Wake The Fork Up®

How to Lose 10, 15 Even 20 Pounds of Fat in 30 Days or Less

By Gary Watson, CSCS

Watson, Gary
Wake the Fork Up®/ Gary Watson.—1st ed.

Includes selected bibliography/references

1. Health, Fitness, & Dieting 2. Nutrition 3. Vitamins and
    Supplements I. Title.
II. Title: Wake the fork UP®.

ISBN: 1505680859

Front cover photos: Tom Zamiar www.zamiarphoto.com
Front cover models: Tiffany Boshers, Gary Watson
Front/back cover design: Killer Covers killercovers.com

Editor: Martin J. Coffee

Printed in the United States of America

For most people, having two supportive, loving parents is more than one could ever ask for. To have three parents has been nothing short of a divine blessing. Dad and Narelle, I love you both and owe you everything.

Mom, your teachings of reaching for the stars and never giving up on dreams have secured me a lifetime of adventure and growth. Phildog, you were the first person to help me understand how health and fitness could change people's lives forever. For this I am eternally grateful to the two of you... May you find some happiness in my continued success as you look down upon me from the heavens.

Never underestimate or underappreciate those who truly support you through thick and thin. While there were many, three must be mentioned, for without these people, none of this could have been possible; Bernie Lecocq, Mark Van Thournout, and Marguerite Walk (Oma). I will forever be in your debt. I am humbled and honored.

Lastly, let me say thanks to my younger sister, Sissy. The first moment my eyes saw you, I begged Mom to take you back to wherever it was you came from. Little did I know my lil sister would become my first best friend. I am so grateful God picked you to be my sister.

One quick note to all of my readers. This book is intended to both teach and entertain. It is meant to carry on a conversation—a conversation that more of us need to have and all of us need to share. There are times when I feel it is necessary to make you laugh and times when I may find it appropriate to compel you to cry. Perhaps you will tilt your head to one side and think, "Wow, I didn't know that." Other times, you may simply say, "Holy shit!" Which leads me to the fact that I do use some (very little) profanity, in this book, when I feel it has a purpose and a place.

Many "professional writers" from the old school of writing will frown upon this, as it doesn't fit within the mold. For that matter, there may be times where this writing seems very casual, seemingly lacks perfect grammar, and doesn't follow the traditional "perfect" writing formula. Guess what? I am well aware of this, and it is by design. I have one goal and one goal only. I want YOU to get RESULTS, once and for all. So, I will do whatever it takes to change your state, and keep you engaged and entertained. In doing so, YOU will get RESULTS like you have never seen before!

As my mentor and teacher Tony Robbins says, "Perfection is the lowest standard on the scale, as it may be attained only for a moment, and then it is gone." So, for those supposed "perfectionists" out there, give it a rest. I, like you, will make mistakes. The master has failed more times than the beginner has even tried. So, if I offend anyone by an occasional misplaced word, a "not so perfect sentence," or even a little profanity here or there, I apologize in advance. And if this still offends the perfectionist in you, that's on you ... not me!

Sincerely,
Gary

CONTENTS

INTRODUCTION 1

CHAPTER ONE: Welcome—Your Total Transformation is Awaiting 15

CHAPTER TWO: The Power of Three..................................41

CHAPTER THREE: My Tony Robbins Revelation 53

CHAPTER FOUR: My Oprah Experience 63

CHAPTER FIVE: George Clooney Confidence with Sleeping Beauty Rest 72

CHAPTER SIX: Scarlett Johansson Curves with Channing Tatum Abs...77

CHAPTER SEVEN: YOUR Seven Super Fat-Burning Hormones 91

CHAPTER EIGHT: Cardio that Rocks—"Moves Like Jagger" 114

CHAPTER NINE: Your Primary Method of Eating & the Power of Three...125

CHAPTER TEN: The Bermuda Triangle of Foods.............134

CHAPTER ELEVEN: Determining Your Nutritional Metabolic Type 165

CHAPTER TWELVE: *Taste of Life: An Intellectual Eating Plan* ....
....174

BONUS—The Biotrust™ Difference: Fat Burning Supplements that Actually Work 181

IN CLOSING 189

SELECTED BIBLIOGRAPHY...191

INTRODUCTION

"We are at our very best, and we are happiest, when we are fully engaged in work we enjoy on the journey toward the goal we've established for ourselves. It gives meaning to our time off and comfort to our sleep. It makes everything else in life so wonderful, so worthwhile."

—Earl Nightingale

Summer, North Avenue Beach, Chicago

I was only one week out from a very important body transformation photo shoot experiment as Slic and I walked up the stairs of the boathouse on North Avenue beach. We had just finished a great day (four hours in 90 degree weather) of beach volleyball, and I was hungry! Not to mention, today was my "super leptin loading" day, and I was eager to put away some fun calories. As we approached the beer and food deck, the first thing Steve (Steve "Slic" Cieslica) said was, "Shoot G-man, whatever happened to the days when we could just walk right up here and grab a seat anywhere we like? We used to own this place." So true, I thought. After all, we had been coming down to North Avenue beach to play volleyball before the new beach house had even been built. In fact, we used to stare at the old broken down, abandoned beach house in agony, as we desperately would have loved a good hearty snack back in the day, so that we didn't have to pack up a cooler, drag it out to the beach, and then back again to the car after four plus hours in the hot sun, giving it our all out on the sand courts. We watched the darn thing (new beach boathouse) being built, and for the first five years or so, we pretty much had the place to ourselves. Naturally, as more and more people discovered the beauty and mystique of the boathouse on the beach, this place became very popular, and for great reason. Some of Chicago's finest musicians perform live music for some of Chicago's hottest beach dwellers at the North Avenue Beach Boathouse. Rightfully so, the days of simply grabbing a seat within minutes of entering were long gone.

No worries, I thought. Although I was very hungry and eager to grab a seat, nothing seemed to bother me these days. As a direct result of my system, I felt so amazing walking and talking in my new body. So while my childish "inner voice" may have thought, "What the hell?" for a second, my mature, real voice said, "No worries." After all, I was feeling 10 years younger than my biological age and looked just as young. My 40-yard dash had found its way back into the sub-five-seconds range. My sports were firing on all cylinders with football (flag football, at this stage of the game), snow skiing, wake boarding, and volleyball being performed at optimum levels with minimum effort. My strength was at an all-time high and my body fat was at superhuman levels. I had gone from a 34-inch waist to a near perfect 30 inches, while packing solid muscle on my chest, arms, and legs. In the last 12 weeks, I had literally lost 31 pounds of fat while putting on 10 pounds of muscle! My mind was clear and precise, proactive and assertive. In fact, I felt like I was 10 feet tall and bulletproof. I had conducted yet another "guinea pig experiment" on myself and was nearing the end of the "set the record straight" plan. More on this plan to come.

I quickly scanned the teeming mob, slapped old Slicster on the back, and said, "No worries, my man; I've got us covered." You see, in the northeast corner, I saw two beautiful, athletic divas sitting at a table of four, all by themselves. Sure there were two other tables with similar setups, but this one was the golden ticket. After all, these young ladies were absolutely beautiful and my mojo was working, if you know what I mean. I had gotten looks, compliments, and surprising conversation startups from beautiful women in the most unlikely places literally everywhere I had gone for the last month. Sure, my body fat was sub-10 percent and I am generally a social person. But wow—the last few weeks had been off the charts. Can you say increased confidence, self-esteem, and hormones? Let's not forget the hormones!

I wasted no time in walking right up to the red- and blonde-haired bombshells and attempted to convince them as to why it would be in their very best interest to share their table with us. To my pleasant surprise, they were more than eager to oblige. We ordered a round of drinks and asked for menus, as Slic and I were hungry as all get up by now.

> *I proceeded to knock back two cocktails, a chicken breast sandwich (sans the bread), two burgers (no bun), and a full basket of Cajun breaded fries, all in one sitting.*

Of course, the conversation and drinks were flowing and before I knew it, we were all back at my place to extend the evening's events. Fortunately, my bachelor pad was only blocks away, in Chicago's beautiful Gold Coast, and it was Saturday night.

We had another drink back at my place, and I even indulged in some all-natural ice cream with the ladies much

3

later in the evening. Turns out good ole Slic had to head back to his place in the suburbs for a prior engagement, so I had to entertain both ladies for the evening by myself. Conversation flowed and the chemistry was amazing between the three of us. Unlike so many other men, often as young as 20, my libido was off the charts.[1] The evening ended and a relationship began as a direct result of my willingness to take a chance and ask strangers if they would care to share their table with us. Believe me—this wasn't always the case with me, as I had spent much of my young adult life overweight and out of shape, with little to no self-esteem to speak of. Thankfully, the tides were turning in my life for the better. Continue reading, as I share more of my journey regarding my transformation.

Yes, I worked off some calories that day with intense competitive volleyball in the hot sun.

> *The truth is, however, that the "caloric burn" wasn't the main reason why I was able to put away over 5000 calories that day. You see, unlike so many other diet and workout plans, I had been using a system in a way that absolutely required me to go "hog wild" with my food intake at least once a week in order to maximize my fat loss!*

That's right, I will say it again—gorging myself on my "super leptin load" day was mandatory for me, in order to lose more body fat. One week out from my 12-week experiment, and I was nearly there. My previous week's measurements

---

[1] Recent studies from the University of Chicago have shown that many young males in their 20's are engaging sexually much less these days. One study also found that these young men's testosterone levels were dangerously low, giving them the same levels of testosterone as someone 15 years older than their chronological age.

had shown a body fat percentage of 8%. What was I the next week? A whopping 6.9% body fat!

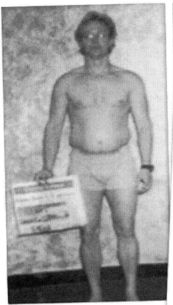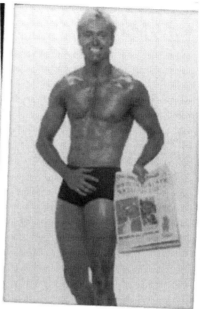

Take a look at the pictures, as they say a 1,000 words and seriously do not lie! Not bad for a guy with poor genetics, as well as limited time and resources, right? I was pleased as well. You see, I had already been in the fitness field for nearly 13 years, and I had helped transform many clients' bodies with very good results. But I had never had a six pack from hell myself before that date in August of 2000. I was definitely on to something magical, and my mind, body, and soul had never felt better. I was in my 30's. As for my mojo, well there was a fine explanation for that as well. Besides the obvious benefits of looking and feeling great, my hormones were off the charts as a direct result of my newfound training and eating formula. Not to mention I had made more money that year than I had ever previously made, and I had just moved into my down-town suite on the corner of Division and Astor Streets, one block from the lake. I was definitely *Looking, Feeling, and*

Being my Best, and I could not have been happier. I was indirectly benefiting in all areas of my life as a direct result of getting my body to shed the fat quickly with ease. Coming from my meager upbringing, I had made it on many levels. I had arrived.

I never, ever had this type of a body in my entire life before this date. Although I had spent the days of my youth playing sports and therefore exercising over 15 hours a week, I was still "fat". In fact, I can remember it to this day, as if it was only yesterday. Growing up in rural Illinois, we literally had one doctor in the entire tiny little town. We also had one dentist. Dr. Koesterer and Dr. Koesterer... they were brothers. So as you can imagine, these two gentlemen had what is known in business as a clear "market advantage." Consequently, Doc Koesterer saw my entire family and the neighbor's entire family, as well as the next house and so on and so forth. In fact, he capitalized on all the local businesses, including our annual school exam. However, when I got to high school, Dr. Koesterer decided to bring a sidekick for my freshman year. He brought a gentleman who would assist in his examination by taking our body fat measurements. Standing in front of me was my friend and fellow football teammate, Robert Brown. Now to my eye, Robert was clearly heavier than me. He jumped on the scale and unsurprisingly outweighed me by nearly 40 pounds. He was, after all, a much thicker, bigger young man than I was. But what happened next not only surprised me, it actually shocked me. You see, Robert's body fat was much lower than mine was.

That is to say that while he outweighed me by nearly 40 pounds, he had less fat on his body than I did (certainly by percentage). In fact, I was so taken aback that I demanded the gentle-

man measure my body fat again. He confirmed that Robert had 13 percent body fat and I had 19. Convinced that this guy had no clue what he was doing, and me not being educated in this phenomenon at the time, I continued to tell myself that there was no way that I was that "fat."

After all, I was a whopping 142 pounds soaking wet. How the hell could I be FAT?

I would have this experience happen to me several times again, until I finally started to realize that there may actually be a phenomenon where one can be over-fat, but not over-weight. Guess what? There is and I was in fact skinny fat as a young child and teen. Even worse was that most of my body fat lay right smack dab on my waist, low back, and love handles. By senior year, it had become so bad that I asked my track coach, Coach Hendog, "Coach, what do I do to get rid of these love handles?" Coach smiled at me as only Hendog could do as he said, "Use them, Watts! Be a lover, not a fighter." We both laughed and I went on to keep that waist fat for another 16 years.

Even worse, however, was that by age 20, I was no longer skinny fat. I was just flat out fat! Consequently, I developed asthma, frequent bouts of bronchitis, and had the energy and self-esteem of a three-toed sloth. In other words, I felt lost and alone, fat and unworthy. It was a terrible time in my life, although I used every source of soothing method I could think of... food, alcohol, and social extremes to distract me from solving my problem. The more wrong food I consumed for my body type, the more bad food I craved. The more beer I drank, the more estrogen my body produced, and the fatter I got. The more I trained my body with the wrong types of exercise, the less energy I ultimately had. Little did I know I was only contributing to throwing my seven super fat-burning hormones into an incredible imbalance at record speed with all of these soothing methods as well.

The more I pretended not to be affected by this with my friends, the more broken I felt inside. Again, like so many others, I used every soothing tactic I could think of to avoid the obvious... I was not looking, feeling, and being my best. In fact, in college, we referred to any guy with a big gut as a "boiler." I was referenced as a "three-toed boiler man" on more than one occasion. And while the guys and I have always picked on each other in a loving and joking manner, the truth was that I never enjoyed this label. In my mind, I was an athlete, a healthy person, a leader and not a follower in health and wellness. In reality, I was sadly mistaken. I had been carrying around unhealthy levels of fat for over a decade and it was beginning to take a toll on my mind, body, and spirit.

So when I share with you my story of how I finally accomplished world-class fat loss and ripped abs to boot in 2000, I want you to know that I am a real person with real challenges much like you. I want you to know that I have failed many more times than I have succeeded. I was eating all the wrong foods for my body type. I was training in the wrong manner and I never, ever had a mental map to follow. That is, until I decided to grab the bull by the horns and educate myself in the best way available. I surrounded myself with the very best and learned from them as much as I could. I then tested each and every protocol on myself and others, fine-tuning along the way. Outside of my guinea pig experiments, I have maintained ripped abs and a body that looks, feels, and acts 10 plus years younger than I actually am for the last 14 years and it feels amazing.

This journey for me has been my life's work and when I finally learned to Wake the Fork Up® in my road of life, nothing has been more rewarding. Sharing my programming with others and watching them get similar results has been one of the most fulfilling experiences of my life.

Truly. So, when you ask me if I think YOU can achieve similar, if not better, results than me, my answer is absolutely YES. So how did I do it? What are my secrets? Have I been able to replicate these results in times to follow?

The answer to your questions are all here in this book. Yes, I have had the privilege and opportunity to create, travel, and enjoy many experiences above and beyond my wildest dreams. And yes, I continue to have amazing chemistry with my beautiful girlfriend. Specifically, on to my body metamorphosis... yes, I have transformed my body over a half dozen times since, each time getting better and better results. Better yet, my results came faster and faster as I perfected my system, year after year. In fact, for the photo shoot for the cover of this book, I produced these amazing results in three weeks. Now mind you, I did not have nearly as far to go for this picture, as this photo shoot did not follow one of my crazy self-inflicted "experiments" to debunk myths in this industry.

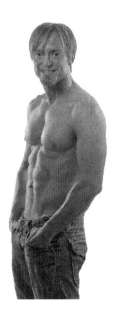

Now, I know what you're thinking, "But Gary, you are a fitness professional, and you stay in great shape all the time." Sorry to tell you this, but I am not a bodybuilder, and I am not a fitness robot. I live a very blessed, diverse, and often stressed life, just like you. I have allowed myself to get more than a little out of shape, while performing "guinea pig" experiments with my body, for your benefit. Not to mention, my genetics are marginal at best when it comes to ripped abs and bulging pecs. Yet, to my great satisfaction and pleasure, I have been able to continue replicating fantastic results, time and time again, overriding my genetics. Even better, my clients have reaped all the same benefits, oftentimes even faster than I did!

Case in point—Geri Levery from St. Louis had always struggled with her weight following the birth of her two beautiful daughters. As Geri says, "Something changed in my body after having my children. It seemed like nothing I used to be able to do worked for me anymore." To make matters worse, like so many women during pregnancy, Geri had put on twice as much weight as she had anticipated with her pregnancies. The result? She ended up being heavier than she had ever been in her life. Even worse, she found herself craving foods in a manner she never remembered experiencing before. After years of battling the ups and downs of many of the "popular" big industry promoted weight loss programs with little to no success, Geri came to me. As I consulted her on the details of the *Wake the Fork Up®* program, her eyes and ears perked up. "Could this be true? Could I really lose this unwanted body fat once and for all, even after all these years?" she thought. Geri was in her 40's now and was really starting to believe that her best years might be behind her. Maybe this was just a symptom of the aging process? How would she ever find the energy to take something like this on, at this stage? All these questions popped into her head as she began to read about my programming.

Then she did something that she will never forget. She said, "Hey why not? Why not take a chance and just try it for three weeks and see what happens?" Much to her surprise (and none to mine), here are her results. Over 50 pounds lighter from her heaviest weight, she has a renewed outlook on life! And it was much easier than she ever imagined. She obviously lasted longer than her three week "trial period." Take a look at her outstanding progress.

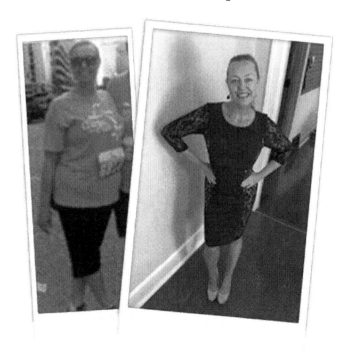

To learn more about Geri's story, go here:
waketheforkup.com/success/

Wanna know what it truly feels like to have the body, mind, and soul of a superhuman? Wanna feel like the sexiest person on the planet as you walk across a room? Wanna look better in a bathing suit than any other outfit you own? Does walking into your office with the confidence of a Fortune 500 CEO, ready to kick ass and take names, interest you? It's all yours and more, if you take a moment to step into my common sense corner and *Wake the Fork Up*® people. Seriously, at least 50% of all the media hype you see, hear, and read about this industry is total, utter crap.

You have been lied too, cheated on, and, even worse, living a very unhealthy life for far too long. Don't waste another day listening to the over-advertised, under-researched, and industry-manipulated sales pitches of the modern day media frenzy we call the "health and wellness" industry. Literally millions of dollars of research and marketing is being manipulated, year after year, to misguide you in order for them to make a buck. You deserve to know the truth, the whole truth, and nothing but the truth once and for all. You deserve to *Wake the Fork Up®*!

The Guinea Pig Experiment

This particular experiment referenced above was to show emphatically that "all calories are not created equal," and that "any type of exercise would do" would in fact not do. This is the old "eat less, exercise more" theory. For 12 weeks, I consumed processed foods (boxed, canned, frozen—you know the foods on the shelves in the grocery stores in the middle of the store), fast food, "diet foods," "low fat" foods, and all the "low calorie" mass marketed foods that were supposedly good for me. I was careful to weigh all my meals for caloric value. I never went over 3100 calories daily, even counting calories consumed in drinks (juices, fancy coffees, etc.). I also did only Low Intensity Training (LIT) for three hours a week. When I started the program, I was at 12.9% body fat at 171 pounds. That means that I had roughly 22 pounds of fat on me and 149 pounds of lean body mass. At the end of 12 weeks on this old formula—calories in versus calories out—I measured in at 23.1% body fat and 182 pounds. This put my fat mass to lean body mass at the following; 42 pounds of fat and 140 pounds of lean body mass. In other words, in less than three months, I added 20 pounds of fat (nearly doubled my pounds of body fat) and lost nine pounds of muscle! What happened the next 12 weeks was even more astonishing. I consumed the exact same amount of calories (calories in), and worked out the exact same amount of time weekly (calories out). But this time,

I ate only the very best, metabolically active, pro-hormone inducing, insulin friendly foods.

For my training, I fused High Intensity Interval Training with both my cardio and resistance workouts. I also manipulated various protocols like periodization, movement tempo, iso lateral movement, and density. Now, I ate exactly 3100 calories a day and trained exactly three hours per week. The exact same amount of calories and exercise time as the first three months. However, at the end of the second 12 weeks, my measurements came in at 6.9% body fat and 161 pounds. That's a mere 11 pounds of fat with a whopping 150 pounds of muscle on my body. I will say it again, I lost 31 pounds of fat while gaining 10 pounds of muscle! The old standby, "eat less, exercise more" (calories in vs. calories out) was a big crock of shit, folks! Don't even get me started on the crazy mood swings, cravings from hell, decreased libido, and overall lack of self-esteem I experienced while on the first 12-week program. At times, I felt like a mad, crazed drug addict looking for my next fix as the sugar, trans fatty acids, and estrogenic compounds started to take over my system. That's how bad the food cravings were for sugary, trans fatty foods. My hormones were also tanking rapidly as I was only doing LIT (low intensity training) in the first 12 weeks of exercise. Bad news Magoo!

Part One

CHAPTER ONE

Welcome—Your Total Transformation is Awaiting

"Never doubt that a small group of thoughtful, committed citizens can change the world. Indeed, it is the only thing that ever has."
—*Margaret Mead*

If you haven't guessed by now, this book experience will be like nothing you have ever imagined. Not only is it power packed with loads of valuable, never seen before secrets, but wait for it...you will actually want to and enjoy reading it. To make things even better, it is packed with beautiful images, valuable graphics, and entertaining video links tailored specifically with YOU in mind. This isn't your everyday "scholastic writing formula" that literally can bore some folks to tears three paragraphs in. Some of you know what I mean. No offense to anyone out there that chooses to stick to that good old formula (as I have many friends, who have written books and done just that). It is simply not the box I choose to be placed in, however. And while we are on the subject, statistics show that less people are taking the time to read a book from cover to cover, although e-books, seemingly, are increasing overall readership for the first time since 1991, because of the many options people have when choosing a device to read on (smartphones are a big proponent of this). While this trend is encouraging, this is why I am doing all I can to make this both informational and entertaining for you.

A Drive Down Memory Lane

Thank you for taking a positive step towards discovering the secrets to losing body fat fast, getting ripped abs, and achieving a nice tight booty. Overall, just looking and feeling your best, in the most effective, efficient manner, once and for all. Like so many others, you have most likely reached a point of frustration, total confusion, or simply a state of curiosity at some point in your life. A state of body and mind where you feel incomplete. Perhaps you feel as if you have come to a crossroads of sorts... a Fork in the road of life. Perhaps it is time for you to make the right turn in life and Wake the Fork Up?

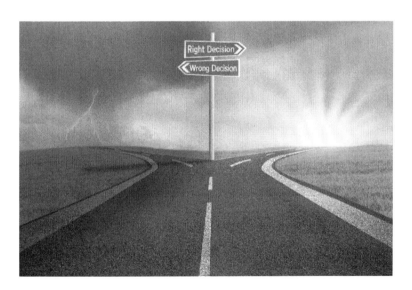

Let's pretend, for a moment, that your body is a car you are driving, fueled by the food you eat, and piloted by your mindset (your navigation system). In other words, visualize yourself as the car, heading on a trip. Perhaps, right now at this moment, you may feel as if you are on a road in your life where you are yearning to find the direction that will finally give you the answers and results you have been seeking. You have traveled the road of dead ends long enough; a treacherous road with long winding curves, and confusing road blocks around every corner. Dark desert highways with no street lights to guide you and no signs of a solid clear direction. Maybe you feel like the driver on a cold winter night, driving through the mountains in a -10° blizzard. With no snow tires and less than 10 feet of visibility, you must traverse long winding curve after curve. Continuously accelerating up the mountain only to brake the next mile, to slow back down, just so you don't crash off the cliff. You know, the kind of driving that gives you white knuckles, because you're squeezing the steering wheel so tight. Or perhaps your drive takes the long, boring flat lands of the Midwest, with little to no change whatsoever, mile after long boring mile.

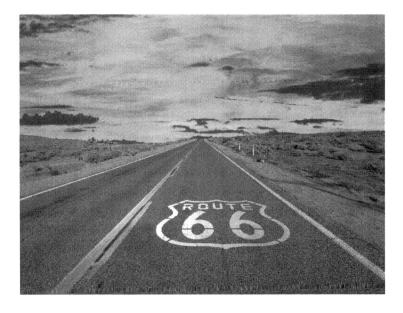

The road changes so little that you literally feel as if you can take your hands off of the wheel with little to no consequences (of course this is not true, yet so many people have done this with their lives/bodies for so long that the consequences have steadily snuck up on them year after year). Or maybe your journey has involved all of these roads plus more, one wrong turn after another, ending up in *"Nowhere Land on Out of Shape Avenue."* Regardless of the road in life you have taken up until now, I assure you that your journey is about to become crystal clear with road maps and signs that will produce red-hot life-changing results. Results that are not only attainable, but also sustainable. In other words, results that you can both achieve and maintain. Not the typical "weight loss" programs that give you some results that never last. You know what I am talking about, so don't make me write out the statistics of those who fail over and over on the scam programs. Instead, let me commend you for your path-seeking ways and assure you that you will not have to look any longer. Because, if the path/road you are seeking will allow you the gift of walking, talking, and breathing in your sexiest, healthiest, and leanest body ever for a lifetime, then you have come to the right place, my friend. *You have finally reached that fork in the road that will change your life for the better, once and for all, just by making the right turn.* So, open your eyes, perk up your ears, and start your new journey NOW. There is no better time than the present to get started in the right direction. Take control of your internal guiding wheel once and for all. Grab ahold with both hands, put your pedal to the metal, and *Wake the Fork Up!*®

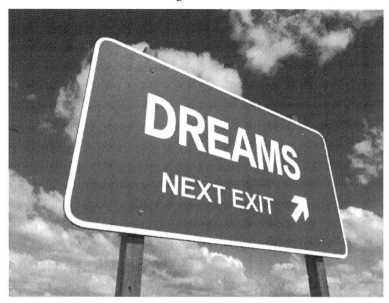

Make no mistake, your journey will involve some planning and an initial small investment in knowledge, preparation, and practices...in YOU. But can you imagine deciding that you were going to take a road trip cross country and doing little more than jumping in your car and taking off..."head west, my good man!"? Seriously, pack up your friends and/or family. Jump in the car. Stop off at the nearest gas station (which happens to only sell diesel fuel, and you're driving a vehicle that uses 93% high octane unleaded fuel), and fill up your tank. Forget about the tire pressure, auto fluids, windshield wipers, etc. Not to mention a navigation system and head on down the road? After all, you did come across this killer advertisement that suggested all your prayers would be answered if you just headed out west. So, off you go, into the wild blue yonder with no worries in sight. That is until you're 100 miles into your journey and realize not only is your car not handling well, but you have no idea where the hell you are or even if you're heading west at this point. I realize this sounds ludicrous to most of you, and yet this is basically what many people often do when taking their journey to a leaner, sexier, healthier body and mind. They literally start a new fad program that they heard about from an unreliable source with no plan at all. Sure, they are told that they will need to exercise x amount of times weekly, eat less of y, and drink more of z, but they actually haven't taken any time (made an investment in planning for the journey ahead) that allows them to truly create a successful fulfilling journey. Your **Wake the Fork Up**® system will finally teach you, once and for all, the three simple steps to not only plan your journey, but more importantly how to arrive there in style.

What makes me so confident you will succeed and who the heck am I? How can I feel so confident that **Wake the Fork Up**® will finally be the spark that ignites your fire, you ask? The life-changing information that transforms your body, mind, and soul once and for all? What makes my programming and commitment to you so much better than all the rest? Who am I to offer you advice? Why the hell am I so confident that YOU can do it? Well, let me tell you, my friend, this confidence didn't just blow in my ear like a cool summer breeze on a perfect evening, while hanging out on the back porch swing, sipping on some lemonade. And it wasn't something that I was just born with either. No, I don't have the "IT" factor, as they would say. In fact, chances are, my genetics, upbringing, cultural experiences, and education were nothing that extraordinary or different from many of you. The photo on the left is what I looked like in college, after allowing myself to fall completely into the abyss, out of shape at nearly 34% body fat. To the right is what I looked like after implementing my program that eventually led to this book. The funny thing is, I am literally almost twice my age in the picture to the right as I was in the photo on the left. If I can do it, so can YOU!

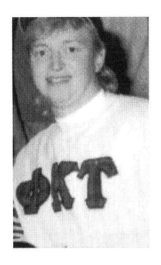 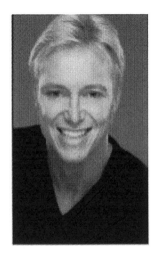

In other words, I have taken a wrong turn and driven down the wrong road before, much like many of you have. I know what it is to be fat, frustrated, and broken on the inside. Yet I have also spent a lifetime studying the best of the best science with some of the greatest leaders in this field. I then turned myself into your personal lab rat to thoroughly test each and every idea and protocol that I will introduce you to. And of course I plan to share every piece of information available to ensure you get the very best results with your top three secrets.

Secrets such as how to instantly start burning up to 300% more fat today. Or increase your natural growth hormone (a powerful fat-burning hormone and muscle shaper/toner) by up to 2000%, with one sneaky adjustment. I will teach you, once and for all, how to eat specific to *your* body's needs. It is NOT like ANYTHING you have ever done before. Yet before I share these life-changing secrets with you, I feel it is necessary to share a little about myself. After all, I wouldn't expect you to simply take my word for it, as you have possibly taken the word of so many other so-called qualified experts before. Let's face it, in today's corporate, profit-driven environment, there are more scams and so-called celebrity "experts" trying to sell you useless information than there are fish in the ocean (or so it would seem). We have all seen it time and time again. Some celebrity or so-called "authority figure" claiming to have found the answer to all your questions wrapped up in a pill, drink, cream, or gadget. They are stating how this hugely endorsed (massive money being paid to the celebrity) product or program is the reason why they achieved such fabulous results. In other words, these so-called experts in the field are nothing more than overpaid celebrities endorsing a product that, quite often, they never even use. They are no more of an expert in the fitness, fat-burning field than I am an Emmy Award winning actor (let's get real folks, as I'm no Robert De Niro). It's a joke people, and frankly it is the wealthy corporations/media trying to dumb you down to sell a product, and it burns my butt that so many of you fall for it hook, line, and sinker. These corporations manipulate the media, much research, and even our government. I call them the "Dumb It Downers," as they constantly do all within their power (and they have a LOT of power) to turn you into "Get By Gals and Get By Guys." People that they can manipulate and distract, so you don't have to think for yourselves. They need you to be a "get by gal or guy" so they can make sure you keep feeding them all your hard-earned dollars on consumption in the form of products, food, clothing, medicine, and health care visits. So they keep the machine going while your health and wellness continue to suffer with their hyped up half-truths. To top it off, you get a smaller bank account, while theirs just gets bigger. So please allow me the liberty and privilege to share with you a little bit about me and my experiences in this ever popular field of healthy, fit, and sexy living, and why I know I am qualified to be one of your new leaders.

....My Revolution of Evolution....

I have had the pleasure and challenge over the last 20 years of working with literally thousands of people that are just like you in many ways. Not to mention, I personally suffered from many of the challenges you are currently experiencing. Consequently, I have learned many approaches, techniques, and methods regarding this subject over the last two decades.

I have studied, read the works of, observed, and even worked alongside some of the world's top leaders in the self-improvement industry such as: Bob Greene (Oprah's Trainer), John Abdo, and Bill Phillips...Tony Robbins, Wayne Dyer, and Zig Ziglar... Dr. David Jenkins, Dr. Joseph Mercola, Dr. Brenda Watson, Dr. William Wolcott, and Trish Fahey. These folks are literally world-class leaders in the elite teachings of our topic of interest—looking, feeling, and being the very best YOU! So, I didn't just pull all of this world-class information out of the clear blue sky. I studied the very best, as I became one of the best in this field. I revised and refined each and every case, and I practiced and taught these principles on client after client. Understand?

Before doing all this, I became a *Kinesiologist* by receiving my degree from the University of Illinois, Champaign-Urbana (home to the nationally acclaimed Human Kinetics publishing house). I studied and mastered all the requirements and exams to become a Certified Strength and Conditioning Specialist (CSCS) (the premier certification with the nationally accredited National Strength & Conditioning Association), and I continue to keep up with all my CEUs to stay current with Distinction. I committed hundreds of hours and tens of thousands of dollars to graduate from the world-renowned Anthony Robbins Companies Mastery University to learn and master the finer art of being a better coach. Through 20 plus years of experience and countless hours, I have finally come up with a fail proof, fat-burning, body-transforming, and total power mindset system. Not to mention, through years of running one of the most successful personal training companies in Chicago, I have had thousands of individuals come to me for answers in this area of focus. Many of whom have paid me over $5000 a month to get them in the best shape of their lives (that's $5000 per each individual). With each client, experience, and intensive study, I found a new opportunity to test the waters of success. With each challenge, I created new solutions for them. The great thing for you is, as a result of their persistence and my passion, I have finally come up with a system I feel is fail proof when it comes to turning YOUR BODY into a lean, mean, fat-burning machine.

> *I do not tell you this to impress you... rather, I tell you this to impress upon you that I have placed years and years (well over 10,000 hours[2]), dollars upon dollars (well over $300,000), and study after study into my system to help guarantee you finally succeed at your goal!*

Specifically, with regard to your physical transformation, I am confident that my program is not only attainable (something you are able to accomplish), but it is also sustainable (something you will be able to maintain). This is because it finally teaches you the truth on healthy, sexy weight/fat loss. The kind of body transformation that your body not only desires, but rewards you for, time and time again. The kind of

---

[2] In his book *Outliers*, Malcolm Gladwell suggests that it takes 10,000 hours to become an expert at anything.

body recomposition that, in many cases, actually allows you to eat more of the great tasting, healthy, whole foods that your body naturally wants. The type of total transformation that enables you to enjoy your life and all that it entails in the healthiest, happiest, and sexiest shape you can ever imagine!

So, I want you to know that this quest, for me, is not a fly-by-night, quick fix scam that gives you temporary water-weight losses or even worse, muscle loss. No, I'm not some celebrity endorsing some quick fix scam product that doesn't know jack about what I'm selling. Again, you see it every day on the television, internet, and radio, but you know that the ONLY reason they are saying they use or like the product is because they are literally receiving hundreds of thousands of dollars, or more, to falsely suggest such things.

> *"A lie can travel half way around the world while the truth is putting on its shoes."*
>
> —*Mark Twain*

Your "Wake the Fork Up" Call
Half-truths and Flat-out Lies

Did you notice that Tiger Woods wasn't driving a Buick when he crashed his SUV into the tree outside of his home (you know, the night his wife allegedly did not chase him down their driveway, swinging a golf club, as a result of his constant cheating with other women)? He had been endorsing Buick for many years prior to his crash. Yet, he was driving a Cadillac. Or even more recently, during the 2014 NBA Finals, when LeBron James had to leave the game for performance impeding leg cramps. Someone from Gatorade actually tweeted, "Had LeBron been on Gatorade® instead of Powerade®, the cramping wouldn't have occurred." This is not what was said verbatim, but it is what was implied (actual tweet, "We were waiting on the sidelines, but he prefers to drink something else."... "The person cramping wasn't our client. Our athletes can take the heat."). The only thing is, he was drinking Gatorade®! What? You mean LeBron James doesn't drink Powerade® during his games? He's been seen everywhere from the Internet to print ads, to billboards, to television claiming, loud and proud, that Powerade® is his athletic drink of choice. Lmao, come on people, Wake Up. He says that crap because he gets PAID millions of dollars to say so, period. Guess what folks, many of those people you see in the fitness infomercials you watch didn't get their bodies by using the products they claim to be using, either.

Seriously, I have worked alongside some of these folks, and they didn't get their bodies using the gadget, pill, or program they claim to have used. I don't want to name names, but the same type of story that I used with the Tiger and LeBron examples are rabid in this industry.

I'm not getting compensated by some big corporation to sell you a bunch of BS. I'm a real guy who went to college to become a Kinesiologist, a Certified Strength and Conditioning Specialist, a coach, and leader in THIS INDUSTRY. I'm just a normal guy that has been actively working my butt off in this field of expertise for 23 years and counting. I'm not the biggest guy in the gym, and I'm certainly not a professional bodybuilder with blessed genetics. I'm just an average ordinary guy that has achieved extraordinary results as a direct outcome of using the exact techniques and principles I am about to teach you. Sure, I have made my share of mistakes along the way, and I am far from perfect. Yet, I am happy and healthy, and I truly feel 15 years younger than my actual age. I walk the walk and talk the talk. Understand?

*Because of these reasons and thousands of sat-
isfied clients, I know that this is the Real Deal.
And when you take the time to fully understand
and follow my Wake the Fork Up® system, you
will turn your body into a Lean, Mean, Fat-
Burning Machine with Brad Pitt self-esteem
and Sofia Vergara sensuality!*

This program has been so successful with past participants that some determined individuals were able to accomplish outstanding results in as little as three to six weeks with liter-ally minutes, not hours upon hours, of invested work time per week. Take Rick O'Neal from Tampa, for example. Rick came to me as a seasoned exerciser who had tried many programs before attempting *Wake the Fork Up®*. In fact, he jokingly admitted that he was a bit of a Beach Body® junky, as he had literally tried the majority of their programs. *Insanity, T25, P90X, P90X2...* he tried them all.

*And in all fairness, Rick said, and I quote, "I
had a fair amount of success with all of these
programs, although the results varied depending on which program. But I had never experienced the results I achieved while using the
Wake the Fork Up® program. Not only were
my results better, but they were much faster
than even I had ever imagined. It was nothing
short of unbelievable."*

These were his results in literally three weeks' time. No exaggeration, no BS, no lie. Real People, Real Results, Really Fast!

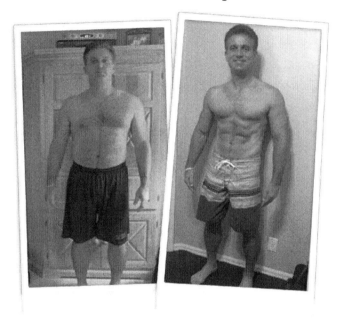

Rick Lost 13 Pounds of Fat in three weeks — Simply
Amazing
To learn more about Rick's journey, go here:
waketheforkup.com/success/

Or how about Pamela Abitua from Chicago?

*Pam came to me with that last 5-10 pounds of
body fat to lose. She reported to me that she
basically was eating well and exercising on a
regular basis. But she felt soft and sluggish.
Even worse, she felt hungry all the time. Once
I taught her how to train properly, eat intellectually, and create her mind map, the system
was effortless.*

The results?

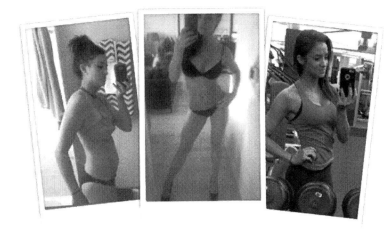

Pamela literally burned 11 pounds of fat in six weeks'
time. Take a look.

Sure, Pam wasn't "overweight" per se by some people's
standards, but she was definitely over-fat for what she
wanted. Look at how soft her arms, abs, and buttocks are in
the first picture. Now take a good look at the next two pictures. Ripped abs, defined shoulders and arms, toned legs,
and a rockin' booty! For more on Pamela's story, go here:
waketheforkup.com/success/.

Let's not forget my journey. While it took me much longer
to get their results, as I made every mistake you could think of
along the way, I eventually learned what truly worked and
what was total BS. I then formulated the system that transformed myself and my test subjects in record time flat. Yep,
I'm not just the creator of this Total Body Transformation system, I am also a client. Take a look at my journey.

Believe me when I say that I was not always the
lean, mean, fat-burning machine you see today
before you. Life is about progress, not perfec-
tion. Keep your focus and attention on the

prize, practice my easy to follow guidelines, and reap the rewards.

There is no system out there better and I am proud to put my name on this program. Ready to take a test drive? Let's read on as I share more valuable information with you.

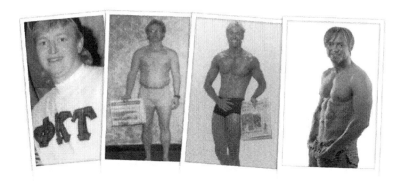

I Lost Just under 60 pounds with this Journey. If I can do it, so can YOU!

You will learn to embrace challenges and incorporate actions that become your *natural flow* instead of fighting the discipline ladder the entire way. You will discover that you are able to eat *more* of the exact foods your body is needing. You will find that less is more when utilizing the right exercise prescription. Another bonus; you may find that your sex life has changed forever!

Now listen, make no mistake; the majority of this book will be teaching you how to burn fat fast and build lean muscle tissue effectively, once and for all. Yet increased confidence and mental clarity will encompass everything you do in life, as a direct result of this journey. This newfound hormonal balance and energy will allow you to become a Casanova/Aphrodite in your own right as well. It is easy enough to do, because as you learn to exercise, eat, and think in this new, exact formula, you will be 90% on your way to being a better lover. And let's face it, not only will you improve all the sexual hormones required for amazing sex, but you will look and feel damn hot doing so once you have dropped some of that very unsightly, unnecessary nuisance body fat you have hanging (literally) around. In fact, did you know that according to many studies, the more fat you have on your body, the less healthy your sexual organs function? It's a fact. Just another benefit to burning fat fast.

> *Think you are too old to get great results? Did you miss the boat? Think again, my friends. My programming doesn't buy into the old adage, "It's just a function of old age."*

Science continues to show us that we can override Father Time again and again when driving our vehicles (bodies) down the right path (waking the fork up). I will share much of this research with you. Still don't believe me? Tell that to Theresa Levy, from Chicago. Theresa came to me as a direct result of wanting to keep up with her beautiful grandchildren. She wanted to be an active part of their upbringing. How do you think she did? You decide.

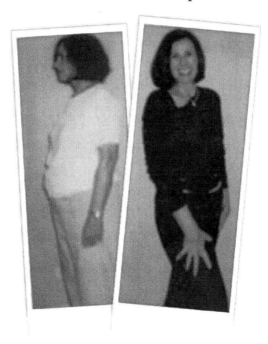

Ace, as her grandchildren fondly refer to her, lost just over 20 pounds in 12 weeks, while increasing lean muscle tone. Beauty has no age limits. Read more about Theresa's story here: waketheforkup.com/success/.

Your "Wake the Fork Up" Call
More Common Misconceptions, Half-truths, and Flat-out Lies

Before I tell you more about this exciting new fat-burning program, I would like to take a moment to address another subject. You and I know that on any given Sunday (or any other day, for that matter), we can find hundreds of "fitness gadgets," "lose weight now pills," or "Hollywood diet" scams waiting around every marketing corner. Not to mention countless Internet and social media ads on how to take this pill or that magic potion to suddenly turn you into a lean celebrity. Or the magic wrap that suddenly makes your breasts look like those of a Playboy bunny? What about that waist wrap that makes you look "slim and toned"? Come on folks, do you really believe any of this malarkey? It's filled with half-truths and lies 99% of the time, and it is very costly as well. It costs you time, energy, focus, health, and of course, your money.

Literally, as a professional in the health and fitness field, it is truly one of the biggest challenges I continue to have within my industry. Jump on the computer and up pops the latest pill to swallow that will magically have you "losing weight" without changing anything else in your lifestyle. Check out the radio, and sure enough, some two-pump chump is talking smack about the latest, greatest "Hollywood diet." Better yet, find yourself channel surfing, and watch some overhyped "guru" tell you how this fitness program or "gadget" is the answer to all the needs of your lumpy bumpy body. It's enough to drive me to drink at times. I can only imagine how it must confuse the hell out of you.

Now, please understand that I realize that these advertisements are oftentimes very enticing. I realize that many of you have even purchased and tried some of these alluring products and programs. And, believe it or not, it's probably fair to say that some of you may have even lost some "weight" on these programs. But here's the trouble... The Thing... THE TRUTH... the majority of weight loss on those types of programs is nothing more than water (fluid) weight. If I had a dollar for every time someone started a program like the ones we are discussing, only to gain ALL the weight back plus much more, I would be earning an 8-figure income. The reason I say this is because NO ONE stays on a "DIET" all their lives, and even if you did, it would eventually catch up to you because it negatively alters your resting metabolic rate (this is the rate at which your body naturally burns calories while you are at rest). And what about those magic pill formulas, you ask? Those magical pill-popping remedies completely tax your central nervous system, internal organs, and adrenal glands. Not to mention that the majority of all supplement companies cut corners and costs by giving you subpar supplements. They rarely give you what they claim to. Instead, they use fillers such as sawdust, wood bark, and artificial colors, preservatives, and sweeteners. This again alters your body's natural hormone production in a negative manner and begins to slow down your body's ability to burn fat efficiently and consistently. Doing planks to get a sexy trim body, or even worse, spending hours on a treadmill... what a joke. The vast majority of these "quick fix" programs rely on water weight versus fat loss. The remaining weight loss, oftentimes, comes from your lean muscle tissue, which is very dangerous. I will say it again—over 90 percent of all quick fix scam products and programs do **nothing** for your lean body mass (muscle tissue), **nada** for your body's natural internal thermostat (metabolic rate), nor **zip** for your body's natural hormonal secretion/production.

If I take your body and clamp you into a human vice and squeeze you, over 60% of your body would be fluids (i.e., water-based fluids, lipids, etc.). So naturally, many people have lost weight on these programs initially, only to regain all the weight back plus MORE FAT than they had before starting their scam plan. This is because they have negatively altered their body's fat-burning engine by screwing up their basil metabolic rate, hormones, and lean body mass percentage. And while we are on the subject, THIS PROGRAM IS ABOUT LOSING BODY FAT, NOT WATER WEIGHT and certainly not LEAN MUSCLE (WHICH TAKES UP LESS THAN A THIRD

OF THE SAME SPACE FAT TAKES UP ON OUR BODIES)!
Observe below and compare lean weight to fat-ridden weight.
They have the same "scale weight," yet their bodies look com-
pletely different due to their body fat composition. Lose the
Fat, Keep the Muscle!

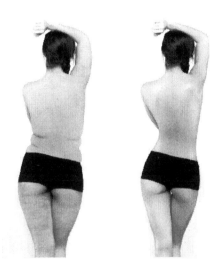

So, while the scale might illustrate one form of your measurements, it is far less important than how your body looks,
feels, and performs. It is much less important than the
amount or percentage of FAT your body loses. This program
is about BODY RECOMPOSITION (more sexy, lean muscle
tissue and less ugly, disease-ridden fat). Believe me, I have
seen many pear and apple shaped bodies lose water weight,
and on the scale, they seemed to be having decent success.
However, when the true test came around, and it was time to
put that bikini/beach wear on, their body's simply looked like
smaller apples and pears. Even worse, their bodies had a
higher percentage of body fat, even though their scale weight
was down. This is not a good look, trust me (as the illustration
above shows), nor does it make you feel great. Their bodies
were not toned, lean, and sculpted like yours will be. We want
confident bodies with tone, shape, and sex appeal. This is the

number one reason why you must do this the right way to ensure you lose fat (not water and, God forbid, not muscle). You must develop tone and increase lean body mass to guarantee that your body becomes a fat-burning machine that continues to stay healthy, sexy, and stunning for many years to come. ***Wake The Fork Up*®** will help you achieve this.

So, take a deep breath and open your mind. You are about to begin a new chapter in life. One that will give you the real deal on these topics once and for all. You are a beautiful, capable, and exceptional human being. Allow yourself the freedom to explore that gift, my friends. Allow yourself to create something great and celebrate life to the fullest. Give yourself permission, once and for all, to ***Wake The Fork Up*®.** Let's celebrate life to the fullest!

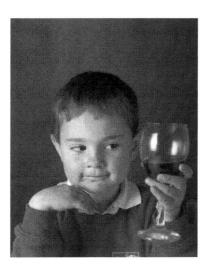

As a part of this celebration, I would like to begin by making a toast. Now, stick with me on this, OK? Let's grab a bottle of your favorite wine. Yes, that's right, as I feel it is time to have a little "whine session." But wait, do not open your bottle or sip your drink yet. I repeat, do not open the bottle just yet! Instead, grab your bottle and head off to the closest mirror you can find in the house. Now, and this is really important...in your whiniest six-year-old voice, look straight into the mirror and repeat after me, but remember, it must be in a whiny, animated, annoying voice:

"Oh Gary, how will I ever find the time to turn my body into a fat-burning machine!?! Whaaaaaa!!!!"

"But Gary, I just want to take a magic pill to turn me into a lean, mean sexy machine!?! Boooo Hooooo!!!!!" LOL!

"It just isn't fair that I actually have to think a little bit before shoving fat storing food down my throat! Big Whaaaaaaaaaa!!!" LMAO!

Or any other lame excuse you have made up until now that has stopped you from producing life-changing results... Remember, excuses are like elbows and buttholes... everyone has them and oftentimes they stink.

Get it out of your system NOW guys and gals. Believe me, these excuses haven't worked for you in the past, and they are certainly not going to work for you now.

> *So, if you truly have a **Belief System** that enables you to use these or other similar excuses, let's rethink this today. Because if your excuses haven't been serving you or your body for the greater good, then those **Belief Systems** are nothing more than a Big Crock of **BS** (bullshit) people!*

Do you honestly think that many others were not similar to you when deciding to take a chance on this program and themselves? Think again. When the Beggs family came to me, they had every excuse in the book, or so it seemed. However, once they decided to give it a try, they were on board hook, line, and sinker. Why? Because every single one of them got results in the first week! Kelly lost four pounds, Nate lost seven pounds, and Scott lost eight pounds in the first week alone... results like this quiet excuses in a New York minute. Nothing, and I mean NOTHING, motivates people more than receiving great results in a short amount of time. Take a look at their success.

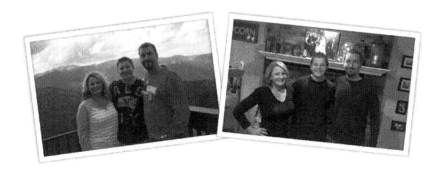

The Beggs Family Lost Over 50 Pounds in Under 12 weeks! Read more about their story here: waketheforkup.com/success/

When Gerold first thought about taking a chance on the program, he also had some reservations. He honestly couldn't remember any other time in his life where he had less available time. He literally almost used that excuse, as so many others have mistakenly done. As a full-time grad student with a full-time job, he literally cringed at the thought of taking on another task. Guess what? He discovered very quickly that taking time for himself drastically increased his overall time management, energy, and even mental clarity. This is because significant science has proven that exercise, when properly executed, improves our brain function. One particular study performed by scientists in Ireland showed that this improved mental capacity was a direct result of exercise increasing

higher levels of a protein known as brain-derived neu-
rotrophic factor, or BDNF. This increase in BDNF doesn't
come from just any old form of exercise. You must exercise at
the correct intensity levels. Once Gerold started using my ***Dynamic Integrated Results-based Training™,*** he was
convinced. Suddenly, this grad student had increased his ability to not only take on more mentally challenging research, but
retain much more of it as well. You can only imagine the rest.
Combine that with Intellectual Eating and the Mind MAPs
and he was hooked. What he realized is that he didn't have
time for excuses. The rest is, shall we say, history... take a look
at his results.

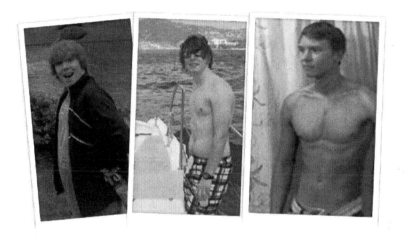

He dropped the excuses and 27 pounds. You can read
more regarding Gerold's story here:
waketheforkup.com/success/.

Again, I encourage you to begin getting over these limita-
tions sooner rather than later. Got it? Good. Not to mention,
your new program addresses all of these excuses and then
some, quite nicely. The ***DIRT™*** workouts maximize results
in minimum amounts of time, all while toning sexy muscle
and incinerating fat. The ***Taste of Life; An Intellectual***

Eating Plan™ crushes cravings and satisfies you with every bite. ***Your Mental Edge***™, cultivating a mindset of excellence, is fun to discover and easy to commit to. Each day on the program, your mental discipline and confidence will increase dramatically, as you will get closer and closer to walking and talking in your Personal Best Body. I have confidence in you and know that you are ready to really get after it with precision, accuracy, commitment, and integrity.

CHAPTER TWO
The Power of Three

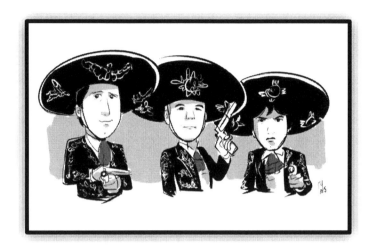

The Three Amigos

"Simplicity is the ultimate sophistication."

—Leonardo da Vinci

Bernie's "That's One"

It was a hot summer night in Chicago, and as I lay down in my bed to take inventory of the awesome weekend I had just had the privilege of experiencing, I heard a very loud and distinct voice from the room next to me. "That's one!" said the B-Man. Rewind, just for a second, to the fall of 1993. I had been working at the world famous East Bank Club on the east river bank of the Chicago River for all of a year and few months by now. I had already taken every in-house exam they had offered me, took on a weekend management position (glorified "we need someone responsible here on the weekends" position), and was one of their leading personal trainers on staff, literally producing 60 plus lessons a week for them (lessons were 45 minutes long). This was both a good thing and a bad thing. Good, because I was one of the trainers in high demand with all the work my little heart could desire. After all, I was a graduate from the prestigious University of Illinois (Champaign-Urbana) Kinesiology Program, and I had passed my CSCS exam from the only nationally accredited association in the industry at the time, the National Strength and Conditioning Association, with flying colors on the first try, even though five other trainers, who had been working there for years, failed the exam, many for the second and third time. I had also gotten my own training schedule and clients in less than three months. This was a personal trainer first at EBC at the time, as they required all new personal trainers to first be a floor supervisor for a minimum of six months before even attempting to get them involved with one-on-one personal management of a schedule, clients, sales, computer work, and all that the job description entails (most would wait over a year to get transferred to a full-time training schedule).

Sure, most every club has a somewhat decent personal training system today, but at that time, EBC was truly one of the elite programs that many other clubs and gyms modeled in years to come. They were ahead of the game, and they needed to be. Their clientele were the most affluent, educated, influential, and wealthiest population of the Midwest. We had the responsibility to move and shake the movers and shakers of the great city of Chicago. It didn't hurt that my first Chicago client was Joy Segal, one of EBC's original investors. She networked me like a blazing fire through a dry forest with the members of the club. I was in high demand, largely due to her. It was a very positive experience, and I generally felt honored with this opportunity. Good to be in such high demand; bad because it can be a formula for burnout. Yet, for any trainer who was new in the industry in Chicago and had hopes and dreams of someday making it "BIG" in the health and fitness industry, it was the place to be.

So, one day, in walks the B-Man (his real name is Bernie, but to me he is the "Bushie Wushie B-Man"—another story for another time). He was fresh out of college, and boy was he green to the city. I mean I thought I was a small town country kid in the city, but man, this dude literally had green shit growing out of his ears... well figuratively, not literally. As I got to know him, it became obvious quickly that he was one smart cat in the area of kinesiology and biomechanics. He was also a little shy, kept to himself, and rarely if ever confronted or challenged me with my often crazy, in your face hypotheses or theories (man, how things have changed, lol). I have never been shy, and forget about keeping to myself. Nevertheless, we quickly became friends, despite our obvious differences. In the months to come, I would pick on him a bit from time to time about his *Green Acres* upbringing (talk about the pot calling the kettle black), and he was always happy to put up with my shenanigans. However, that was until one particular morning in the spring of 1994.

It turns out B-Man had reached the point of no return with his living arrangements in Crete with his parents, and he was willing to tell me about it in no uncertain terms. He was also unwilling to take my shit on this particular morning. All the usual suspects that break a young man at that age were plaguing him... overworked, underpaid, multiple hours commuting in traffic that could make you peel your own skin off, especially on Fridays, and a general sense of just needing to break away from the confines of living under the same roof as his parents (who are amazing people, for the record). So of course I did what any good red-blooded American would do, and I said, "Hey, I have an extra bedroom at my place. Come check it out and see if it might work for you." Well, the very next night, there was a knock on my door and there he was.

Only he wasn't alone—he had also brought his secret weapon, his girlfriend April. I say secret weapon, because unlike B-man, April was extremely chatty, very city savvy, and she was a powerful negotiator. To make matters worse for me, she was petite, beautiful, and smart (think Pamela Anderson at age 20, with a big giant brain). As it turned out, April had gotten me to give Bernie my extra room for one third of my rent, as well as my parking space in the garage, before I even knew what the hell had hit me. When I came to my senses, I did get my parking space back, and what the heck, one third of $475 was still ok with me. After all, his room was half the size of mine and pink, as we would later find out, as we are both color blind. Literally, it was an ongoing joke of our friends, as they never cared to share it with either of us until many years later. And yes, I did say $475, which was ridiculously low rent, even for that time. Not that the apartment was big, but it was clean and freshly remodeled, and it had plenty of space for two young bachelors. And let's face it, Roscoe Village (Chicago neighborhood) was nothing like it is today, but I knew it was still a great deal. Thanks Bob and Des!

So, here we were in this little two bedroom basement apartment, on a hot summer night, and all of a sudden I hear, "That's one!" Now you must realize that B-man is a guy I often refer to as "a man with deep pockets and alligator arms." He is very frugal with his money, and particularly so when it comes to paying ComEd (our local utility company) with his hard-earned cash. So, consequently, one of the first compromises I had to make, as an adult with a roommate, was the fact that our thermostat was kept high in the summer and low in the winter. It was always so amazing to me how this guy could be so "hot" in the winter in the apartment and so "cold" in the summer (the whole alligator arms scenario). Nevertheless, we learned to make it work by having our only box fan propped up in the kitchen, pointed in the direction of both of our bedroom doors, because there were no windows in our bedrooms, and we were desperately trying to circulate any cool air that might be available at night in Chicago. As a result, it was not uncommon for us to both lie in our own beds, after a long day, and chat a bit before dozing off. It kind of reminded me of John-Boy and family saying good night throughout the house every night before going to bed on that old television show The Waltons...."Goodnight John-Boy, goodnight Mary Ellen, goodnight Mama, goodnight Erin, goodnight Ben, goodnight Jim-Bob, goodnight Jason, goodnight Elizabeth, goodnight Grandma, goodnight Grandpa, good night"...well you get the picture.

Realizing we had ended our nightly ritual of screaming from room to room to discuss our day nearly 20 minutes beforehand, I was surprised and a little startled to hear "That's one," at one in the morning. In fact, to be honest, I wasn't even sure if he actually said that or if I had simply dozed off and dreamt such a preposterous thing. So, I lay there for a moment and then started to drift off again...only to suddenly hear, "That's two." Now, I was certain he had said something and I hadn't just imagined it. So of course in true "John-Boy" form, I decided to engage in more conversation. "What the heck are you talking about B-man?" "Oh, you know," he replied with a chuckle. "I don't know," I answered with a laugh. "Oh you know," he persisted. "You know that every night, when you go to bed, that you ALWAYS let out three great big loud yawns before I hear you snoring away." 'What the heck?' I thought to myself. "Are you busting my balls?" I replied. He had one simple answer, "Nope!" We both started laughing. I settled back into my pillow and that was the last thing I remember. The next morning when I awoke to confirm his story, he said that my three yawns were like clockwork every single night, and I was amazed that no one in my family of eight had ever noticed or told me this before. The funny thing was that he claims to have shouted out, "That's three," after my third yawn, but of course, I never heard him. I was fast asleep, as he had predicted. I am a world-class sleeper, thank God. The funny thing is that to this day, I will occasionally catch myself performing this ritual and as a direct result, will say to myself, "That's one," "That's two" and laugh myself to sleep.

Now, you might be asking yourself what this story has to do with the Power of Three? To be honest, I'm not exactly sure, outside of the fact that it reflects many things in my life. Three has always seemed to be a pattern in my life. Not to mention, it is a great true story with which to capture your attention. You see, generally, I have subconsciously used the Power of Three my whole life, in many ways. For example, I have a general rule that I will attempt challenging or uncomfortable situations three times before taking a new approach. I can learn most any information, trait, or skill, as long as it is presented in no more than three different concepts at once. I can multitask better than most, but only if it involves no more than three things at once. I am the third child of six, and my mind naturally chunks things into threes often, even when I am unaware of it. Absolutely true... three is something of an anomaly with me.

Well, it turns out that I am not unique in this way. In fact, I am quite ordinary regarding the Power of Three. You see, many studies have proven this to be the case for many people.

Tony Robbins alludes to the Power of Three in the following way: the mind basically says "One, Two, Three... too many...One, two, three...Too Many...one, two, three...TOO MANY." In other words, our minds generally learn best in chunks of three.

Offer us more than three new concepts or tasks at once and the effectiveness and efficiency of the learning process is greatly reduced. It's not that we are incapable of learning more than three concepts at once; it's simply that our minds do not want to. This happens on an unconscious level for most of us and can become damn frustrating when we are trying to excel at something new. This is why I developed **Your Primary M.E. and the Power of Three™.** My job is to make things as simple as possible for you in many ways. This is why I have designed everything in a method of three to ensure you get the very best experience possible with all the great new information you are going to learn. So sit back and relax—the information will be presented in a manner that allows you to take three small bites at a time. It's all in the design, and it's all about YOU!

Your Primary M.E. and the Power of Three™

Do you still want to know how to burn 10, 15, or even 20 pounds of fat in 30 days? Do you want to know the secrets to having Six Pack Abs and a Tight Sexy Ass? It is a unique system that I have designed specifically for you called your **Primary M.E. and the Power of Three™.** Simply put, there are three very specific identities you will begin to take on regarding the new you—your Primary M.E. This new Primary M.E. will show you, in exact detail, how to slash your body fat in half in six weeks or less with the patented **DIRT**™*y* training method. It doesn't involve hours of boring cardio, and you aren't using some ab gadget doing hundreds of abdominal exercises. This hybrid training method turns all your fat-burning hormones on naturally, while simultaneously resetting and regulating all the fat-storing hormones. In fact, one sneaky trick will have you **burning up to 10 times more fat**, according to a study in *The Journal of Strength and Conditioning Research*. The training secrets are world class, never seen before modifications that torch the fat off of your body. You will have ripped abs, sexy buns, and toned arms and legs in record time.

Your new Primary M.E. will strategically tackle tough situations better than an NFL linebacker. You will literally have the best MAP available to navigate the fastest fat burn ever, with the added bonus of increased self-esteem, confidence, and sexual chemistry. No more fighting temptations and cravings 24/7.

> *In fact, this style of eating has been proven to increase natural human growth hormone (GH) production by 1300-2000%, according to the American College of Cardiology in New Orleans. This is very powerful, as GH is the number one hormone when it comes to having lean muscle tissue and extremely low body fat.*

No more overthinking seemingly complicated issues regarding this quest. Your new Primary M.E. teaches you YOUR specific nutritional metabolic type and exactly how to eat intellectually, once and for all. Guess what? You are not like everyone else. This way of eating is designed specifically for your body type to increase toned lean muscle, while simultaneously burning massive amounts of fat. It also requires you to go hog wild once a week, but in a clever way that actually allows you to burn more fat than ever. In fact, for the ladies, once your body fat reaches a certain level, you get to "super leptin load" twice a week, as you are more leptin resistant than men. In addition, little secrets, like having this specific type of cinnamon right before you eat the "bad" foods, will reduce the likelihood of you storing fat on your treat day. It's true, and it is all in here.

And if turning the dial up to 11 on your pheromones is of interest to you (and it should be), there is one great way to do this within one week's time. You will literally start to notice a massive increase in the admiration you begin to receive just while walking into a room. It enhances your sex fiend machine! Your new Primary M.E. will decrease the Real Age® of your sexual organs by as much as 10 years in six weeks' time. Nothing in this program is what you are hearing from the corporate masterminds behind big media (television, Internet, magazines, etc.) who are supplying you with bogus information. *Your new Primary M.E. will allow you to look, feel, and be your best once and for all. The best part about it....you will learn all of this in Three Simple Steps.*

Your Three Primary M.E.'s—A Summary

Your first success secret is developing your **Primary** **M**indset of **E**xcellence. That's right, the first step to becoming your personal best is to develop a mindset that encourages and strengthens your mission, every step of the way, called *YOUR Mental Edge™.* I'm not talking about looking in a mirror and doing useless affirmations. I'm talking about a solid lifestyle coaching program that will enable you to take on any challenge with ease and enjoyment. This set your mind free method is not like any other formula you have tried before. Through simple, yet specific guidelines, you will quickly develop the three most important aspects of YOUR fat-burning **M**aster **A**ction **P**lan. This MAP will literally get you from point A, smoothly through point B, arriving at your destination (point C) in the best shape of your life. Are you ready for the journey of a lifetime?

Your second success strategy is your **Primary M**ethod of **E**xercise, or second Primary M.E. The secret to literally turning your body into a fat-burning machine is to exercise in this precise, prescribed manner. I'm not talking about spending endless hours on a treadmill or doing hundreds and hundreds of ab exercises. You're not going to do hours of pelvic thrusts, planks, or kegel exercises either.

> *Your newfound way to exercise is a unique take on all the exercise programs you have ever encountered, and the best part of it is that you can do it anywhere (home, office, gym, outdoors). It is an exact science that takes ONLY the very best of several workout techniques and fuses them into a new-age hybrid format called* **Dynamic Integrated Results-based Training™ (DIRT™).**

This hybrid fusion training is literally ground breaking and produces the fastest fat-burning results available.

Lastly, in order to complete your total transformation, you will need to develop your third Primary M.E.—your **Primary M**ethod of **E**ating called ***The Taste of Life; An Intellectual Eating Plan™.*** The third way to burn body fat most effectively is to eat the right foods, at the right times, in the correct amounts, specifically for YOU.

YOU have a Nutritional Metabolic Type specific to YOUR needs, and it is different from many other folks. YOU also have a specific Eating Opportunity Window. So do not think this is yet another "blue plate special" one-size-fits-all routine.

This certainly isn't your basic calories in versus calories out routine (and while we are on the subject, we do not count calories here, gang). That approach never creates a fat-burning metabolism that allows you to discover your leanest, sexiest body. And believe me, this is not a diet program. That very word makes me feel ill. Have you ever taken a moment to really look at the word? **DIE**t...hmmm, something to think about. Unlike the typical diet approach, this program allows you to eat plenty of healthy, delicious foods with built-in "super leptin loading" days that actually help you to burn even more extra fat. The key is knowing how and when to do this. I will teach you this, step by step, in an easy to follow format. But again, people, please, please, please understand—this is not some mainstream formula to help you lose weight that you have seen and heard before. The program, ***Taste of Life; An Intellectual Eating Plan™,*** not only tells you what to eat for YOUR specific needs, it also tells you exactly when and how often. And guess what? It isn't four to six small meals a day every two to three hours. This is a totally new, ultra-hybrid way to help you incinerate body fat. And best of all, it is as easy as one, two, three.

There are three weird little tricks to make you burn fat faster than ever; three simple ways to metabolically supercharge your food; three simple ways to make your mind that of a mini-

Einstein. It is all here, crystal clear, and easy to follow.

Put simply, this program will NOT include fad starvation diets, typical workout routines, or directionless instructions that are not practical in your everyday lifestyle. This program will NOT have you running on treadmills like a lab rat for hours on end. This program will NOT have you looking in a mirror telling yourself "Because I'm good enough, I'm smart enough, and doggone it, people like me." This programs works! Read on as you discover the what's, why's, and how's of your new program in detail. I promise you that this is not Keyser Soze and his *"Usual Suspects."*

CHAPTER THREE
My Tony Robbins Revelation

"One reason so few of us achieve what we truly want is that we never direct our focus; we never concentrate our power. Most people dabble their way through life, never deciding to master anything in particular."

—*Anthony Robbins*

May 2005, Paradise Island, Bahamas

The day had been nearly perfect, as the evening approached with one of the most beautiful sunsets I had seen in years. Kat and Dave had just tied the knot on the beach, precisely at sunset. If I had to guess, they paid extra for that little piece of beauty (in fact, I'm sure of it). Weddings in this part of the world are literally planned in advance to the very minute to guarantee such things, and Mother Nature was more than happy to deliver. Following the ceremony, we all headed to our deluxe outdoor waterfall venue for the real fun…. let the party begin!

After a few drinks, much dancing, and general shenanigans, I found myself sitting at a table with the groom (Dave), friends Steve and Mark, his father-in-law Tom, and two other cats (guys) I had just met that evening. Because I had recently just returned from a trip to the Fiji Islands, the guys wanted to hear about the trip while we rested our dancing legs from our gals. The ladies, naturally, were still out there "busting their moves."

While in Fiji, I attended one of my many intensive, week-long, Tony Robbins Master University programs. During his programs, I have literally swam with sharks, climbed up 100-foot telephone poles and stood on top of them looking out over oceans before jumping off the pole (with a harness), and walked across burning hot coals (that is right, I am a fire walker). His ability to lead a person like me to accomplish amazing feats are not surprising to me, as I am now an adventurous beast. His ability to coach **millions** of people to do the same amazing feats, however, impresses the hell out of me. I mean, this man is by far the most phenomenal lifestyle coach I have ever encountered. And if you haven't seen him, I highly recommend you do, regardless of any preconceived notions you may or may not have of him. After all, he has worked with over four million people, in 100 different countries, over the last 35 years—people such as Nelson Mandela, Bill Clinton, Mother Teresa, and Oprah Winfrey.

Actor Steven Weber, from the television show Wings, attended one of Tony's events. He described his experience of the UPW seminar as follows: "Being somewhat of a skeptic myself, I didn't know what to expect...every second was worth it. It was an experience like no other I've had, and Tony is, to put it mildly, extraordinary. I've never seen anyone walk the walk like this guy, have never witnessed someone able to match and exceed the energy of an audience of 6,000 inspired, hopeful people."

Oprah Winfrey showed up to one of his events expecting to stay for "an hour or two." Twelve hours later, she was still there, long and strong, taking notes from this master.

Andre Agassi, Hugh Jackman, Eva Longoria, Quincy Jones, Donna Karan, and Serena Williams are among some of the other rich and famous individuals who are happy to offer up a testimonial to describe Tony's impact on their lives. And NO, they were not paid to do so!

Still not convinced he may know a thing or two about helping ordinary people develop extraordinary lives? That is not surprising, on some levels, I suppose. You see, I have met three kinds of people, regarding Tony Robbins, over the years—those who have never heard of him at all; those who think they "know him," but have never attended one of his live events; and those who have seen him live. Undeniably, **every single person** I have ever met that has seen him live, **without exception**, came away absolutely amazed at just how extraordinary he is in person. This goes for all the people who "thought" they knew him and many who even thought they would dislike his work. He literally is that freaking good.

When sharing some of my experiences with the group at the wedding, they all consistently came back to one question…"How did he get you and all those people to do these things?" To be honest, he is a master technician that utilizes many advanced training systems and methodologies, but these guys were chomping at the bit for just ONE piece of advice.

So I sat back, took a sip of my vodka and water on the rocks, and said, "Where Attention Goes, Energy Flows."

They all stared at me with their heads tilted to the side, like a dog looks at its owners when spoken to.

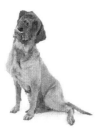

So, I went on to explain some simple concepts on how we all have the ability to transfer energy by applying laser-like focus to any task at hand. This laser focus (attention) produced amazing results via energy transfer (measured vibrations/efforts/actions/etc.) that had been seen in most extraordinary achievements. For certain tasks, it goes without saying, the more attention you give something, the better result you will get. However, we have all experienced being "in the flow" at least once in our lives, and the bottom line is, the energy we are transmitting as a direct result of our newfound focus is vibrating at a level that brings greatness to us through actions, awareness, opportunity, and execution. When you are tapped into this energy, you can literally do things that most people can't even comprehend. This is when things seem to just come easy to us. Not that we haven't worked hard preparing our mind, body, and soul for the event, but man, once we are in the flow, we are unstoppable. Once we Wake the Fork Up®, we conquer fears, capture moments, and seize the prize! Amazingly enough, this attitude completely overpowers and overflows into everything else in our lives as well, not just our health and wellness. Believe me, once you have achieved this goal of becoming a leaner, sexier, healthier being, many other things in your life are gonna shape up as well. And it all is reliant on your thoughts, your attention, and your ability to find the energy necessary to succeed. If for some reason you think your thoughts and energy don't have any effect on your life or others, think again.

Back at Paradise Island, I gave the guys some very simple examples of my statement and then decided to try out a little experiment. You see, the hotel Atlantis has a world-class casino. And while none of us were big gamblers, we all planned on spending a little time in the casino after the wedding reception had come to a climax. After all, we had all taken a four-day weekend, and we were all planning on making every minute count. So, I "pumped them up" on the fact that positive energy would invariably have an effect on a social game like craps. For those of you who have never been at a craps table, this is by far one of the most social games one can play while gambling. The basic premise is that a group of people stand around a rectangular craps table and either bet with the person rolling the dice or against the person rolling the dice. Every person at the table will have the option to throw the bones (roll the dice) when it is their turn, should they choose to. If you do not wish to roll, simply pass the roll to the next person. Should you ever find yourself walking through a casino and you hear roars of praise and celebration, more than likely there is something going good for the majority of participants at a craps table. I have personally met more people at the craps table than even at the pools in Vegas. And I love getting my pool on while in Vegas.

Based on the fact that we, as a group of six, could make up half of a table's players, I was convinced that we could not only have a great time playing the game as a group, but I was also convinced that we could get the other half of the table to come to our viewpoint of the rolling (as in bet the same way we were, **with** the dice roller) by simply channeling our attention in an extremely positive way and sharing that energy with the group. This meant that no matter what a dice roller did—win, lose, or draw—we would always keep our conversation very positive, clap, and encourage each and every dice roller. We would also set the standard of communication with the stick man and his two counter dealers at the table as well. No negativity whatsoever, only positive energy. Our attention and focus had to be unified, in alignment, and on point. "Who knows," I said, "maybe we can even make a little money." However, I warned all of them to only bet with money they intended to spend as entertainment. After coaching them to a level of excitement, it was time to conduct my little experiment.

So, we headed into the casino and walked past a few full tables. No, no, no....hmmm, YES, I said. There was a table off to the far south corner with only a few people and perhaps the minimum bet was low enough for me to take the newbies. Yes, 10 dollar minimum, and we could easily fit all six of us at the table, not to mention I could take my favorite position at the table as well, immediately to the right of the stick man. This position has always given me a little advantage with my throws, as I have a systematic way to toss the dice that limits the degree of freedom the dice "ideally" should take. We got to the table. I was very proud of the guys, as they all immediately started being positive and supportive of the three other players at the table. The rolls were just ok, but we all continued to support each other and the "strangers" at the table, even when their rolls cost us some money. I did have the newbies follow my lead on a system that pulls your winnings off the table in a manner to minimize any risk of losing too much too fast. So, it made it a little easier for them to stay positive through thick and thin.

Thirty minutes went by and, all in all, my group was just about even on our money investment in the game. In other words, we had paid nothing to get free drinks and entertain ourselves (a win for social gamblers like us). The table crew really started to take to us, and the slumping postures and quiet demeanors became tall, sociable table men and one beautiful woman, who were actually cheering for us as we had a few minor victories (after all, the house money is not theirs, they get paid whether we win, lose, or draw). The attention (and intention) of making this table an absolutely positive experience for all was 100% on track. Also, every single person at our table was betting **with** the dice roller and not against them. A few other gentlemen slid up to the table as we continued, although they were at opposite ends of the table from where I was standing, and I did not get a good glance at them as my focus was on the player rolling the dice. And just like that, the "IT" factor happened. One of the original three guys at the table (not one of my crew) got HOT! Our energy was already so positive and strong that we were peaking at a near maximum enjoyment level as a group, so when Shane hit six points (wins) in a row, quite honestly, we were not surprised. Elated, hell yes. Surprised, not one bit.

However, we did suddenly get a little louder, as he was "on a roll" and now our break-even play was reaping some real financial rewards—cash money, G, cash money! The guys were amped, and I was getting pretty damn excited myself. Chants like "Stay Hot Shooter" and "Shooter, shooter, shooter, COME on SHOOTER" were flying with abundance. We were on point and loving every minute of it. So, after the sixth point was won by our shooter, and the dealers were busily counting, dividing, and handing out all our massive winnings to each individual, I actually heard a "Shush" from the other end of the table, to the opposite side of the stick man (a player whom I could not see at the moment). Before I could glance over to see who on earth could be at our table not enjoying this experience, the shooter had the dice back in his hand and it was time to roll, baby. So, my focus went straight back to Shane, and this dude rolled the bones for another 23 minutes solid. We all banked off of his dice rolling like Warren Buffet's kids in a candy store ordering up a cart full of **Chocopologie by Knipschildt** (the world's most expensive chocolate at $2600 a pound). Shane had a roll of a lifetime, and we all reaped the rewards of it big time.

Now, as I stretched across the table and looked past the stickman, I looked down to see who the hell "shushed our table."

> *It was none other than NFL superstar quarterback Donovan McNabb and two of his friends. By this time, he was smiling as he put his finger to his lips and made a "shhh" sign to me with a wink. I looked him dead in the eye and said, "McNabb, I don't tell you how to run an offense, don't you tell me how to run a craps table."*

He simply smiled, as did I, collected all his winnings, and walked away. As we all counted our money, and the frenzy came to a halt, we looked back behind us and there were rows and rows of people collected behind us, feeding off our energy and focus. There were literally over 10 rows of smiling, happy people on the side of the table my crew was on. They were all so excited to simply be around us and our experience, even though they themselves had not won a single penny in our game. The other side of the table, you know, the side with the NFL superstar celebrity...well, they, however, had simply one small row of people. I laughed my butt off, all the way to the bank (the chips to cash exchange at the casino), on that realization.

But, get this if you will. I ran into Donovan's friend the following morning, at the gym, as he walked up to apologize for Donovan trying to "shush" us. He stated that Donovan was afraid that people would recognize him and that they would all start to ask for his autograph and ruin his anonymous fun. He also told me that Donovan made a nice bit of coin at our table, as he was betting with much larger amounts of money, and therefore reaped much greater returns. I told the friend no worries, as he didn't bother us. I also stated that I didn't notice anyone asking for his autograph near our table and laughed. The friend told me, "Yeah, surprisingly no one must have recognized him." I simply smiled and proceeded to whip the snot out of myself with a **DIRT**™ workout that awed most of their guests and, again, smiled to myself. Not only did we get everyone to have a great experience at our table and make lots of money...but NO ONE EVEN NOTICED DONOVAN McNABB WAS AT OUR TABLE, BECAUSE THEY WERE TOO BUSY TRYING TO BE A PART OF OUR ENERGY." Yep, an NFL superstar had total anonymity at our table. How did this happen? **Simple, where our attention was going, everyone's energy was flowing**, even the spectators in the casino. While it was a very informal test of this theory and it was only for fun, I assure you, I have created very similar results with many difficult challenges in my life, and so have thousands of other folks just like you. It was an incredible experience to witness and be a part of.

So while there are literally hundreds of things Tony has taught me over the years, your first step in developing your Primary Mindset of Excellence is to practice the theory of "Where Attention Goes, Energy Flows." One of the best ways to direct your attention is to develop your **M**aster **A**ction **P**lan (**MAP**). Remember we talked about this earlier in the book? In order to get to where you are going, you must first know where you are currently, and have a solid idea as to where you want to go. The best way to do this is to apply **SMART** goals towards where you are and where you want to be. In other words, take specific, measurable, attainable, realistic, and time measurements NOW on where you are in your healthy, fit, sexy life. Then sit down and come up with **S**pecific, **M**easurable, **A**ttainable, **R**ealistic, and **T**ime-sensitive goals for where you want to be. For example, you currently may weigh 210 pounds, with a body fat of 33%, a waist line of 40 inches, and a sex life that seems minimal at best. Take a good honest look at these facts and jot them down in the starting section of your **A-MAP**.

Next, forgive yourself for traveling to this place and immediately start focusing on where you want to go. "I will lose 40 pounds on the scale, while slashing my body fat by 50%. I will cut my pants size down to a 34-inch waist. I will have a firm, fit stomach and a chiseled chest. I will become more adventurous and energetic with my lover and begin having fun, fulfilling sex at least three times a week." Or perhaps you are a size 12, with low back pain, and get out of breath walking up stairs or playing with your children. For you, it may perhaps be a statement like, "I will run a 5k with my kids for their annual charity run, lose three dress sizes, and finally take that adventure travel trip I have always dreamed of, in three months. I am a work in progress and will take a step forward each and every day to ensure I will reach these goals within 12 weeks. I will revisit these goals often to hold myself accountable."

> *These are SMART goals, people, and these are necessary. Saying "I want to be fit and beautiful" is not gonna cut it. It has no specificity, no real form of measurement, and no timeline towards attainment.*

So, the very first thing you must do is get your MAP designed so you know where to focus your energy, like a laser, once and for all, to become a lean, mean sexy machine.

CHAPTER FOUR
My Oprah Experience

"The future depends on what you do today."

—Mahatma Gandhi

Your "Wake the Fork Up" Call

I first came across this quote in 1999 when reading Bill Phillips' best-selling book, *Body For Life* (although, I do not know if he created it) and it has resonated with me ever since. "If you Fail to Plan, then Plan to Fail." It is a really simple concept, and yet so few people practice it with any consistency, and consequently, achieve minimal results, at best. You must take the necessary time to learn the proper techniques, approaches, and practices to create your ultimate MAP (**M**aster **A**ction **P**lan).

I will simply say it one more time. "If you Fail to Plan, then Plan to Fail." You must make a little effort in the beginning to truly understand the principles and practices that will allow you to create the most successful **M**aster **A**ction **P**lan (MAP) in order to truly succeed once and for all with your journey towards becoming a confident, capable, hot mess of a specimen!

Now, it's not a MAP that involves a magic pill, a goofy gadget that burns fat from your hips and thighs, or a special fruit juice from a tropical rainforest. And it isn't the same old

63

adage, "eat less, exercise more, and get disciplined" either. These programs never work long term, and oftentimes not even in the short term. It does involve learning how to make YOUR body and mind work best for YOU, once and for all. And even if you have already tried dozens or even hundreds of other programs, I can guarantee you that this program is completely different than any other program you have ever come across. It is the best, most cutting-edge information available to date, and it will literally change your life. These top three secrets involve information that is so imperative in your journey to becoming a lean, mean, sexy machine that without learning these secrets once and for all, you risk becoming just another statistic. I have seen it change thousands of ordinary folks into extraordinary leaders. Leaders in life with glutes of steel and ripped abs. It can happen for you too. Of this, I am confident. Sure, there may be some information you have heard before on some level, but I assure you that in this book, you will discover the secrets to new techniques, strategies, and lifestyle habits that will make you feel superhuman.

So, right now before we do anything else, let's make a basic MAP of exactly where you are now and where you want to be in 6-12 weeks. You can refine this after reading more, but for now, let's at least get some basics down. This Master Action Plan (or MAP) is YOUR navigation system that ensures YOU get to where you want to go, while keeping you off the side road made of dirt and potholes that can destroy even the best journey. So right NOW, fill out the beginning and end points of your MAP, point A (where you are now) and point C (where you want to go). MAP B will be your ACTION MAP that allows you to make all the right moves to arrive at point C. Your B MAP is what the Fast Track covers. MAP B will also illustrate where you are along the way and if and what types of changes you may need to make to keep yourself on the best road possible, so that you arrive in the time frame you have designated.

Remember, life is ever evolving and dynamic in nature, and filled with crossroads and turns. Develop your map now so these little surprises do not cause you to crash along the way. If you already completed this earlier, simply transfer your info here now.

Your A-MAP

A-MAP: Realistically, where are you now?
> *Pictures: Front, Back, and Profile*
> *Clothing Sizes:*
> *Scale Weight:*
> *Body Fat Percentage:*
> *Body Measurements:*
> *Eating Habits:*
> *Exercise Habits:*
> *Mindset: clear, foggy, or somewhere in between*
> *Energy Level:*
> *Athletic Event/Achievement:*
> *Other:*

Your C-MAP

C-MAP: Realistically, where do you want to be in 6-12 weeks?
> *Pictures:*
> *Clothing Size:*
> *Scale Weight:*
> *Body Fat Percentage:*
> *Body Measurements:*
> *Eating Habits:*
> *Mindset:*
> *Energy Level:*
> *Athletic Event/Achievement:*
> *Other:*

"There are two types of people: those that talk the talk and those that walk the walk. People who walk the walk sometimes talk the talk, but most times they don't talk at all, cause they walkin'. Now people who only talk the talk, when it comes time for them to walk, you know what they do? They talk people like me into walkin' for them."

—*Key talking to DJ in the movie <u>Hustle and Flow</u>*

Now, I can lead you to the water my friend, but it will be your job to do the drinking. I don't mind if you talk the talk, but you best be walking while you're talking. And yes, I have done a lot of "walkin' for you," but now it's time for YOU to walk the walk. Because even if I had the time (which I don't), I couldn't do it for you any more than I already have in my programming. The rest will be up to you. So, let's take three minutes to take your first step in the right direction. Let's have you take at least three measurements today that tell us where we are on the MAP in the here and now. Just pick any three measurements on the chart. Do it NOW!

So, what are you waiting for? Why did you not take the time to do this first step? You can blame it on any number of things: time, convenience, other people, or circumstances. You can tell me any excuse you want that blames the problem on someone or something else. But as Zig Ziglar said, "People who *are* the problem never recognize that *they are* the problem. They are in complete denial. They actually think denial is just a river in Egypt. I've discovered that in 100% of situations, **no exceptions**, people who won't take step number one never take step number two." So, take your first step now.

Great Job! Now you are walking the walk. Keep it up.
Three more minutes. Name three goals that you want to
achieve in the next six weeks. Make them tangible, measurable goals that are very specific to your desires, and make them
realistic. "I just want to feel healthy" is not a tangible, specific
goal that can be measured accurately. "I want to lose three
inches off my waist circumference. I want to lose 10% body
fat within six weeks. I will fit in a size six dress in two
months." These goals are very specific, measurable, attainable, relevant, and time-bound. These must be **SMART**
GOALS.

Lady O and Bob Greene

I have never been more meaningfully reminded of this very
fact than during my experience with Bob Greene (Oprah's
trainer) and Oprah. When starting out in the fitness field, I
began working at the prestigious health club known as EBC
(East Bank Club). Not only was it "the club" by virtue of its
sheer presence, staff, and equipment (over 400,000 square
feet with over 1,000 pieces of equipment, 20 tennis courts,
three basketball courts, squash, racquetball, kinesis wall, spa,
beauty salon, three restaurants, pools, studios, business center, etc.), but it was also the home to some of Chicago's biggest
movers and shakers. One, in particular, was none other than
Oprah Winfrey. You see, Oprah had always attempted many
avenues with her struggle for weight loss throughout the early
years and had even worked with my boss at EBC at the time,
Dave Smith. Now, Dave was an excellent manager...friendly,
approachable, reassuring, and attentive to all the crazy needs
of his "wild n' crazy bunch" of trainers back in the day. After
all, we were all young, dumb, and full of...well you get the picture. But, as a trainer himself, Dave was subject to the powers
that be in corporate America and their formula. He had to

push clients in and out as much as possible, as this was the training formula that the corporation demanded. The more training sessions he and his trainers were able to bill out per month, the more stable his job was, and this was also reflected in his pay.

He had the knowledge and skills to be an excellent trainer, but he lacked a certain mindset when it came to the client. He was missing the lifestyle coaching aspect that every great leader must have to make the connection with their students. I will never forget my first interview with him. When asked why I felt most of EBC's clients would want to work with a trainer to begin with, I enthusiastically blurted out 10 specific, goal-oriented, achievable reasons as to why I could and would help change their lives for the better in a timely fashion. His response stunned me in the beginning, but as I soon learned what EBC's real personal training program was about (making money), his approach became clearer to me. His view on it, as my manager, was that most people loved to work out with his training staff as a measure of sociability, comfort, and relationships. 'What the,' I thought to myself. 'How the heck are we going to measure that?' Now, don't get me wrong; I have developed amazing relationships with many of my clients over the years, and being an active part of their lives is often a great benefit of this. But make no mistake—people need specific measurable goals that are relevant to their specific capabilities (attainable) and have a specific beginning and end (time bound) when wanting to really transform their bodies.

Not only had Dave missed this with his staff, he also missed it with his "Golden Goose" opportunity while working with Oprah. You see, Oprah had worked with Dave for a short period of time, but unbeknownst to him, she wasn't about cushy long-term training relationships to "feel healthy," even if that is what she said. Because in a very short time, she fired him. Before I knew it, Bob Greene was showing up with her, her bodyguards, and anyone else she wanted to bring to the club. For the record, she was the only person, to my knowledge, granted permission to bring an outside trainer (non-EBC employee) to EBC to train with. For those of you that don't know the rest, Bob focused in on her like a big game hunter and got her in the best shape she had ever been in. How did he do it? What made him so special? I know Bob personally and have even had the opportunity to work along-side him. He flew me out to his home on Fischer Island, just off the coast of Miami, to encourage me to work for him back in the day. He is a very intelligent man with a great attitude on life and a reassuring combination of confidence and calm-ness that is infectious to be around. But most importantly, he gave Oprah **S**pecific, **M**easurable, **A**ttainable, and **R**elevant goals that she could and would accomplish within a very spe-cific amount of **T**ime. The results were, of course, great and the Golden Goose made Bob a very, very wealthy man. Bril-liant Bob, brilliant I say! **(SMART GOALS)**

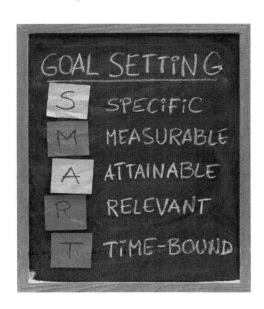

Take a moment and write down three SMART goals right here, right now.

THIS IS ESSENTIALLY THE BEGINNING OF YOUR C-MAP—YOUR UTOPIA!

1st SMART goal:_____

_____

_____

2nd SMART goal:_____

_____

_____

3rd SMART goal:_____

_____

_____

Beautiful work! Now take a picture of this page and make sure you look at it at least once every day. After all, it is YOUR MAP, your chosen path...your destiny! Do it now, and embrace your new journey.

Remember, a famous Harvard University study once tested the reason why a group of graduates varied so much in their success, many years later, when they reconnected.

Twenty years after the research had been completed, those who actually wrote down their SMART goals (only three percent of them) achieved greater wealth and success than the remaining 97%. Set these goals with purpose and passion, write them down, snap a picture of them, look at them, and revisit them...they are much more powerful than you know. Great job. You are well on your way and that wasn't so hard, was it? In fact, you are already closer to succeeding than you think.

If you are truly serious about taking these maps to an expert level, shoot over to waketheforkup.com/programs/ for your personalized Master Action Plan MAPS with Smart Goal guidelines and more. You can find it all here in our *Wake the Fork Up®* **Your Mental Edge**™ program.

CHAPTER FIVE

George Clooney Confidence with Sleeping Beauty Rest

"Our minds influence the key activity of the brain, which then influences every-thing; perception, cognition, thoughts and feelings, personal relationships; they're all a projection of you."

—Deepak Chopra

Step Number Two—Retrain Your Brain

Your subconscious mind is constantly communicating with your conscious mind whether you are aware of it or not. This internal dialogue can literally sabotage your new body transformation goals in no time at all. From internal fears to past experiences and failures, this process can be deeply rooted inside of you, waiting for the perfect opportunity to tell you without hesitation that "you will fail." This happens for many reasons, such as past failures, ego identity, fixed percep-tions, and a general lack of consciously taking responsibility for one's actions. As previously mentioned, Big Corporations prey upon you with this knowledge and often do all within their power to encourage you not to stray out of the yard and explore new things. They want you to be "get by gals and get by guys," so they can tell you what to do. Predicated upon fear and their basic formula of wanting you to care about what oth-ers think of you (more than what you think of yourself), con-form to social norms, and stay in your comfort zone, these false perceptions and constructs contribute to self-sabotage. In fact, when people view their abilities as fixed (fixed perceptions), they were more likely to be anxious when they face challenges, according to a 2007 study by social psychologist Jason Plaks. This anxiety often leads to folks subconsciously talking themselves out of achieving goals, by making excuses as to why they will fail prior to and during the challenge that lies ahead. The trouble is, rarely will a self-saboteur actually admit to self-sabotaging. This is because they often are not consciously aware of it, although many of their friends, family, and co-workers are. Remember, if your Belief System is not serving you for the greater good, it is nothing but BS (bullshit). Don't let limiting beliefs take control of you.

One great way to overcome this is to educate yourself on such issues and to consciously and consistently take control and responsibility for your life. This will change your perception of your abilities, and you will be well on your way to great achievements. By reading this book, YOU are already educating yourself and by making your MAP, you have already taken responsibility for your life, so you are well on your way. As Anthony Robbins instructs in his famous *Get The Edge Program*, you must change your physiology, empower your focus and beliefs, and change the language that you use. Your MAP has changed your focus and beliefs, and we are about to teach you how to change your language. You are absolutely capable and deserving of reaching and achieving your every desire. You are capable of slashing your body fat in half or more and looking and feeling your best. You are deserving of having more confidence and sex appeal than Heidi Klum and George Clooney. You are on your way to having more energy than most others who are 10 years younger than you. You are capable of remarkable actions that produce an extraordinary life. I know this about YOU, and YOU must know this as well!

To learn how to implement the second secret weapon in developing your mental edge today, head to waketheforkup.com/programs/. This method is super effective and super easy. Once you learn this, you will no longer sabotage your goals.

> *"My father said there were two kinds of people in the world: givers and takers. The takers may eat better, but the givers sleep better."*
>
> —Marlo Thomas

Step Number Three—A Simple Night's Sleep

Being distracted, overstressed, and not in the moment has led to more **dis**ease and **dis**order in your life than you know. Not only does it significantly rob you of precious quality time with family and friends, it also drastically inhibits your body from recovering and healing naturally with good quality sleep every night. This lack of quality sleep wreaks havoc on your work experience, energy, mental focus, and sex life. It practically stops your ability to efficiently burn fat as well. It literally slows down our good hormones and speeds up the bad hormones when it comes to burning fat fast.

According to the US Centers for Disease Control and Prevention, roughly 50 to 70 million American adults suffer from sleep and wakefulness disorders. This lack of quality sleep has been tied to mental distress, depression, anxiety, obesity, hypertension, diabetes, high cholesterol, and certain risk-taking behaviors, including cigarette smoking, physical inactivity, and heavy drinking.

And according to the Journal of Clinical Endocrinology and Metabolism, people who sleep less tend to fall victim to the old adage of the "see food" diet. In other words, they want to eat everything they see!

Not to mention it throws your fat-burning hormones completely off track.

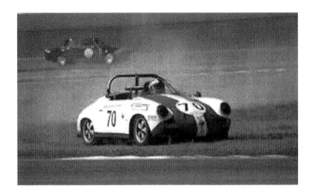

We already spoke about this to some degree, but it is so critical that it is truly one of the key components to the three secret steps. For example, the University of Chicago has reported that young men who got insufficient sleep in their twenties experienced a reduction of testosterone by as much as 15%. This effectively aged them by 15 years! This drop was also accompanied by a massive increase in cortisol, according to a study published in the *Journal of the American Medical Association*. These two hormonal changes alone will impede your energy and fat-burning goals significantly. However, lack of sleep also increases your ghrelin (the hunger hormone), while decreasing your leptin (the I'm full hormone). I think it is time to rethink your sleeping habits, peeps.

"In the past, many people thought that sleep was a waste of time," Dr. Bruce Nolan, director of the sleep center at the University of Miami Miller School of Medicine said. "It was to be avoided. And getting seven or eight hours of sleep was a sign of laziness," he continued. "That kind of thinking is outdated," he said. "We have lots of evidence that getting good quality sleep is associated with a better quality of life."

So how much sleep are we talking about? In general, the studies suggest that a minimum of seven hours allows us to get the quality REM sleep patterns our bodies require. Sure, eight hours may be better, but the crucial point seems to be seven for most of us, regardless of how "special" or "unique" you think your sleep habits are. In fact, researchers at the University of Naples Medical School discovered that people who sleep less than six hours nightly have a significantly shorter life expectancy. The University of Warwick has also confirmed these findings.

In short, you must begin to get a consistent quality sleep rhythm if you have any chance of becoming a fat-burning machine. Once you do this, you will increase good hormones, like growth hormone, testosterone, and leptin, while decreasing fat storing hormones, such as ghrelin and cortisol. The days of not getting quality rest are no more folks. This is how we change this pattern tonight—waketheforkup.com/programs/.

Part Two

CHAPTER SIX
Scarlett Johansson Curves with Channing Tatum Abs

Your <u>Primary</u> Method of <u>Exercise</u> & The Power of Three

<u>There's Something About Mary</u> (1998)

Hitchhiker: You heard of this thing, the 8-Minute Abs?
Ted: Yeah, sure, 8-Minute Abs. Yeah, the exercise video.
Hitchhiker: Yeah, this is going to blow that right out of the water. Listen to this: 7... Minute... Abs.
Ted: Right. Yes. OK, all right. I see where you're going.
Hitchhiker: Think about it. You walk into a video store, you see 8-Minute Abs sittin there, there's 7-Minute Abs right beside it. Which one are you gonna pick, man?
Ted: I would go for the 7.
Hitchhiker: Bingo, man, bingo. 7-Minute Abs. And we guarantee just as good a workout as the 8-minute folk.
Ted: You guarantee it? That's—how do you do that?
Hitchhiker: If your'e not happy with the first 7 minutes, were gonna send you the extra minute free. You see? That's it. That's our motto. That's where we're comin from. That's from "A" to "B".
Ted: That's right. That's—that's good. That's good. Unless, of course, somebody comes up with 6-Minute Abs. Then you're in trouble, huh?

[Hitchhiker convulses]
Hitchhiker: No! No, no, not 6! I said 7. Nobody's comin
up with 6. Who works out in 6 minutes? You won't even
get your heart goin, not even a mouse on a wheel.
Ted: That's a good point.
Hitchhiker: 7's the key number here. Think about it. 7-
Elevens. 7 dwarves. 7, man, that's the number. 7 chip-
munks twirlin on a branch, eatin lots of sunflowers on
my uncle's ranch. You know that old children's tale
from the sea. It's like you're dreamin about Gorgonzola
cheese when it's clearly Brie time, baby.

I love this scene in the movie, and have always appreciated the idiocy that so many people choose to believe about the myth of having ripped abs. Of course, no gadget or program that exclusively trained your abs could or would ever get you ripped abs. And while eight-minute abs may sound appealing to most, simply doing eight minutes of ab isolation exercises will not transform your body in a manner that reduces your body fat to the necessary levels to see "ripped abs." However, the flip side of this is that unlike the other myth, I do not train my abs for hours and hours per week.

> *In fact, I just barely put in over 18 minutes of*
> *direct ab isolation exercises per week. It is all*
> *the other secret training methods that I will*
> *teach you that give me rock hard abs. Eighteen*
> *minutes of abs per week is less than three*
> *minutes a day, people.*

Think about that! Maybe I should make a three-minute abs program, Lmao! Wanna learn how I and so many of my clients got their ripped abs? Well then keep reading ;)

Wanna know the second secret to developing your best fat-burning body ever? This is what we call your second ***Primary M.E.—Your Primary Method of Exercise.*** That's right, the second SECRET to fast fat burning is...wait for it... Exercise! Really? No kidding, you might ask? "Yes, *really, really,*" as Shrek would say. HOWEVER, PLEASE DO NOT THINK THAT I AM REFERRING TO JUST ANY OLD EXERCISE PLAN. The kind of quality fat loss that we are looking to achieve requires much more science than that old, dusty "just do anything" exercise mold that so many have wrongly chosen in the past. Sure, any movement will get you some very small results for a brief period of time, but our goals are those that consist of no small task. That old formula and so many other hyped "new" formulas will not get you ripped abs and rock solid bottoms (neither will the eight or seven-minute abs program ;). Our mission is to help you achieve the best, sexiest, most confident body you have ever had the privilege to inhabit. Consequently, our exercise prescription or second ***Primary M.E. and the Power of Three***™ is very unique, specific, and specialized. In fact, it is so specific and special, when it comes to burning fat fast, while keeping and oftentimes increasing lean muscle, that I actually trademarked this exercise training program. The name of this fat-blasting program is ***Dynamic Integrated Results-based Training***™ (***DIRT***™). So, do not be fooled and think that I am simply talking about yet another "weight lifting" program, body weight exercise plan, or yet another Low Intensity Training program like jogging for hours on end. Those programs are weak and insane.

Dynamic Integrated Results-based Training™ *(DIRT™)*
An Exercise Formula that Incinerates Fat while Toning Muscle

This program is so simple, and yet so powerful, all at the same time. It consist of three steps. **First,** you will learn my patented, secret formula that has **three *different weekly* training protocol systems called *Dynamic Integrated Results-based Training*™**. And by different, I am not referencing the highly promoted "six different exercise DVDs" you see on TV, as they train your body with the exact same "system." My protocols are absolutely different from a scientific approach that maximizes results in the least amount of time, while keeping you safe from injury. **Second**, you will train **three specific muscle groups in sets and blocks which are mapped out over three days**. Three days of **DIRT™** resistance for a minimum of nine minutes a day combined with three days of **DIRT™** cardio for a minimum of nine minutes a day. **Third**, I will teach you, once and for all, the top **super sneaky secrets** to achieving the very best results in the absolute shortest amount of time. The discovery process is fun. The results are amazing. And best yet, it is so simple.

Let's imagine for a moment that your *body* is a *car* you drive in, your *food* is the *fuel* for this car, and your *mindset* is the *road* which you choose to drive upon. Continue to imagine, for now, that you are a big old, rusty Cadillac. Even worse, your Cadillac has a modified, broken down 4-cylinder engine, heading down a highway to "health hell." The body of this car is rusting, and you have low tire pressure. You have no navigation system and, for all practical purposes, are stuck in a rut on the road. To top it off, even if you wanted to toot your own horn for help, you wouldn't because it comes out sounding like a vuvuzela horn.

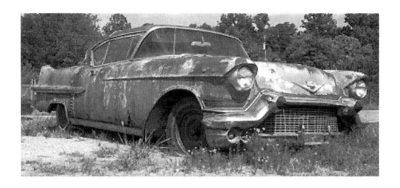

According to wikipedia: Traditionally made and inspired from a kudu horn, the vuvuzela was used to summon distant villagers to attend community gatherings. The vuvuzela is most used at football (American soccer) matches in South Africa, and it has become a symbol of South African football as the stadiums are filled with its loud and raucous sound that reflects the exhilaration of supporters. The intensity of the sound caught the attention of the global football community during the 2009 FIFA Confederations Cup in anticipation of South Africa hosting the 2010 FIFA World Cup. For those of you unaware, the vuvuzela has been the subject of controversy when used by spectators at football matches. Its high sound pressure levels at close range can lead to permanent hearing loss for unprotected ears after exposure with a sound level of 120 db(A) (the threshold of pain at 1 meter (3.3 ft) from the device opening). These horns were banned from many fields and rightfully so, in my opinion, as they are annoying. But enough about that damn horn.

It can be pretty daunting, visually, when you take it all in, and I wonder just how many of you would jump in this car and head on down the road. Would you pull up to your friend's place in this car? How about heading to a business gathering among your work colleagues in this car? Would you feel safe and secure taking this car on a long, cross-country trip, or racing it down a drag strip? Would you invite others to ride in your car? Think about it.

Now, imagine if you will, that you are about to get into an Aston Martin V-12 super sleek, sexy sports car.

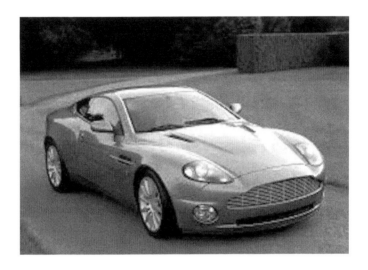

This 48-valve 60° engine produces 450 bhp and 400 ft-lbs. of torque. It is controlled by a drive-by-wire throttle and a six-speed Electro-hydraulic Manual Transmission. The standard Vanquish model had 14.0 inch drilled and ventilated disc brakes with four-pot calipers, ABS, with electronic brake distribution.

The V12 Vanquish's appearance in the 2002 James Bond film *Die Another Day* (driven by Bond who was being played for the final time by Pierce Brosnan) earned the V12 Vanquish the number three spot on the list of Best Film Cars Ever.

This is a beautiful, finely tuned machine. Sure, you can go from 0 to 60 in four seconds flat. Yes, your Pirelli p Zero Corsa tires are at a perfect 34 lbs. of pressure. You have a horn that sounds beautifully elegant and powerfully seductive. You have provided the car with the best fuel available and, of course, your navigation system is top of the line.

You are driving and arriving in style every-where that your heart desires. The funny thing is, however, that you don't even need to toot your own horn, because people see you from miles away, as you turn the corner filled with confidence and mystique. You, my friend, are a mystery that most simply cannot take their attention away from. You have arrived in class and style. You have reached the fork in the road and taken the correct path, once and for all!

This is literally what your Primary M.E. and the Power of Three™ and **DIRT**™ does for the human body. The results are amazing, and the benefits are endless.

Dynamic Integrated Results-based Training™ *Resistance Training* *(DIRT*™ *Resistance Training)*

Dynamic Integrated Results-based Training™ incorporates—you've guessed it—THREE different training styles or protocols all together within a one-week period, as opposed to the same old workout style/routine day after day, week after week. Each workout systematically addresses and challenges ALL of the tough fat deposit areas on the body, albeit a little differently for each. Each trouble zone gets hit hard every week, therefore accelerating your fat loss results in record time. This expeditious process occurs because science tells us that there are several factors outside of our individual genetics that contribute to fat storage in our troubled zones (belly fat, hips and thighs, back of the arms). No worries, as my hard work, experience, and scientific research have you covered to maximize all of these trouble zones.

In general, as you place various degrees, modes, and styles of exercise upon your body's system, many wonderful biomechanical processes take place. One ideal style of exercise is weight bearing resistance training. When it is introduced to the body, the natural response is an increase in strength, lean body mass, and resting metabolic rate. This is, by far, one of the most superior ways to transform your physique. However, with traditional forms of weight or resistance training, this effect can quickly diminish as your body naturally begins to adapt to your training protocol or routine. Eventually, your workouts produce less results, and the only way to keep the positive, transforming results coming is to continue to increase the workloads. And while you may be able to do this in the beginning, you will eventually reach the dreaded plateau. Not to mention your joints, tendons, ligaments, and muscles will most likely begin to ache as you continuously attempt the next big lift. Of course, you could always increase your workload by exercising more and more each week, but will you really want to or be able to? This can actually diminish your progress as well. After all, the very fact that you are reading this book is because time is very valuable to you. The good news for you is that I have developed a better way that considers the need for appropriate weight bearing exercise while respecting the time constraints that pervade each day. But if you think my **DIRT**™ program is simply another "weight training program," think again. Nothing could be further from the truth.

Why DIRT™ Works

Those of us in the know have always used various forms of periodization to "confuse," "shock," or "surprise" the body. And as a result of many studies showing better results with periodization (changing your training program at regular intervals or "periods"), many periodization programs were developed. The problem is that most individuals simply are unaware of the power of periodization, and they continue to do the same old routine over and over again. Before you know it, no matter how hard you work out, you just can't seem to achieve the same results you used to be able to. And for those who "think they know periodization," particularly with resistance/weight training, most people stick to a very simple periodization protocol. It generally looks something like this for resistance training. Endurance training consists of 2-3 sets of 12-20 repetitions at a low to moderate intensity level for some designated amount of time (4-12 weeks). General conditioning consists of 2-3 sets of 8-12 reps at moderate intensity for approximately 4-12 weeks. Strength periodization generally consist of 5-8 repetitions at a high intensity for the program's assigned time frame (4-12 weeks). And some even do a power periodization for 2-4 reps at high intensity for some specific amount of time (perhaps 4-12 weeks). That's it, as they ONLY focus on resistance loads and repetitions. And the worst part about it is that MOST people never break out of using only one of these periodization programs. Consequently, not only do they start to see less and less results as the program goes on, but they also often get injured from overuse syndrome. In addition, they trip up their natural hormone release system as a direct result of training incorrectly.

Or you have the folks who say throw out periodization all together. You know, the group that claims to only do "functional" movements with no structure, plan, or system.

I have met with many of these "groups" over the years who were trying to promote "over 3000" different "functional" moves, declaring they haven't repeated a workout in over three years. Considering one of the lead "functional" training gurus is over 30% body fat, as are many more from this group, I think I will say the best program lies somewhere in the middle. Gang, it is perfectly ok to expect some great "vanity results" (looking freaking awesome naked) as a reward for all the hard work you put in. You can be the most "functional" person in the gym and easily look like a lump of potatoes under your clothes. It's bogus at best and damn tragic at worst. You are not here to put in the work and get little to no body transformation/recomposition changes. So, don't let them confuse you. You must have a system that is both simple and specific to YOUR needs, wants, and desires. Forget all the rest of it. Got it? Good!

Lastly, many folks out there who do not understand this will try to argue this point. The majority of all "weight lifting," "resistance," and cardio programs out there never work your *super fast twitch muscle fibers.* Some barely work your fast twitch. For many, their traditional "strength training" primarily works their slow twitch muscle fibers, regardless of what you might have thought. Sure, you may be fusing some fast twitch fiber recruitment, but super fast twitch fibers...forget about it.

This is yet another important reason why "traditional" workouts are just not cutting it. You are basically rejecting your body's natural physiology by not working the other half of your muscle fibers (super fast twitch). You think it is any wonder why our fast twitch and super fast twitch fibers drastically disappear as "we age"?

We stop pushing ourselves with vigorous, fast twitch movements like climbing monkey bars, racing from tree to tree playing tag, and just a general sense to push and challenge our bodies. I am not saying you should be climbing monkey bars, but I am saying you damn well better learn to start recruiting your fast twitch and super fast twitch fibers, if you want to move forward. Come on now. **DIRT**™ changes all of this for you, guaranteeing that you never fall into a plateau and that you always train to maximize fat burning while keeping lean muscle.

"Insanity: doing the same thing over and over again and expecting a different result."

—Albert Einstein

Your "Wake the Fork Up" Call
Workout Insanity

Let me repeat—the fact is that most programs only use one form of training protocol and/or periodization to begin with, without you even knowing it. Even many of the very popular programs you see on the Internet and television today. Sure, those "popular" body weight training programs address metabolic training, but where is the true strength training? Believe me, in less than three weeks on that program, you will NEED more than simply your body weight for true strength training benefits that continue to provide lasting results and sustainable fat loss. Not to mention, these popular programs do not practice many of our secret weapons. This of course limits their effectiveness. Do not worry—we've got this covered for YOU.

Secondly, those who do attempt to use periodization only manipulate the resistance loads (amount of weight lifted) and repetition ranges (amount of repetitions completed). And, this is very important, they stick to these periodization periods *way too long*, even if they are doing it right (most are not, however). Now, we know that traditional periodization programs can produce much better results than those that only do the same routine over and over. But unlike traditional forms of training, ***DIRT*™** constantly changes your type of exercise strategy by manipulating tempos, ranges of motion, rest intervals, repetition ranges, exercise formats, functional range of motion, and resistance loads. Even better, it does all of this during the same week. Not every 4-12 weeks, like the old plans do. We actually turn the old recipe inside out and complete an entirely different style guaranteed to get you ripped in record time. Out with the old and in with the new. This helps to guarantee that your body never stops receiving the much-needed and well-deserved results you are seeking.

But, it gets better. With ***DIRT*™** training, we work you at the exact right intensity as well, guaranteeing that your FIT formula is ideal for burning fat while building shredded muscle. Believe it or not folks, we never, ever exercise over 45 minutes in any one setting. This is absolutely critical, and precisely where so many go wrong. We also never take rest intervals longer than 90 seconds, again ensuring you get the absolute BEST FAT-BURNING results ever. We also recruit and work your fast twitch and, most importantly, your super fast twitch fibers. This is absolutely crucial to your success. Making sure we train the right way and for the correct amount of time, we get an increase in the natural production of super hormones like growth hormone, testosterone, leptin, and irisin, all while reducing insulin, cortisol, and ghrelin. In other words, not only do you produce more of exactly what you need with this style of training, but you also effectively address hormones that don't serve your body, such as excess estrogen, cortisol, and insulin resistance that causes so many to be overly fat in these troubled areas.

Unlike traditional resistance training, we stand and incorporate some form of lower body movement and stability factor into nearly 90% of all exercises. This requires your body to work much more while doing all exercises. Even a bicep curl or tricep extension becomes a compound joint movement, for example. It also increases your overall muscle activation tremendously, which burns more calories in a much shorter period of time. And because this added movement involves the largest muscle groups in your body, your natural production of growth hormone skyrockets!

Lastly, and most importantly, **DIRT**™ takes three of the very best training styles for burning fat fast and keeping and toning lean body mass to a new level. It literally manipulates Metabolic Training, Lactic Acid/Time Under Tension Training, and Explosive Strength Training. That is to say, these three styles train your body energy systems differently. Understand? Most other programs only use one energy system and therefore limits your results very quickly. This maximizes your super hormones significantly. These three styles of exercise combined in this precise format will literally allow you to get results in minutes instead of hours. You will see increased growth hormone, testosterone, leptin (all the lean muscle building, fat-burning hormones) and decreased cortisol, ghrelin, estrogen, and insulin (all the fat-promoting hormones). Trust me, there is no better style out there, period.

DIRT™ will have you looking like Scarlett Johansson and Channing Tatum in no time at all! And the best part about this ground breaking training style? You can get it instantly, today, by simply going here: <u>waketheforkup.com/programs/</u>. You think I am kidding you about how unique my training system is? So did Rick O'Neal from Tampa... that is until he tried my system and got the best results of his life. This is because not only is this system completely unique by design, but it also is the best format on the planet for increasing your Seven Super Fat-Burning Hormones.

Remember, you can read Rick's story here:
<u>waketheforkup.com/success/</u>.

CHAPTER SEVEN
YOUR Seven Super Fat-Burning Hormones

"Happiness is not a matter of intensity but of balance, order, rhythm, and harmony."

—*Thomas Merton*

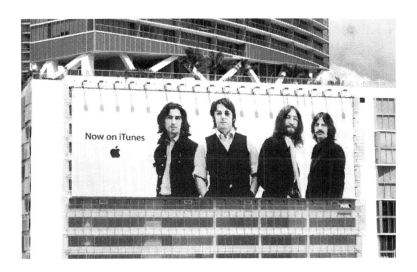

THE FAB FOUR
GH, INSULIN, LEPTIN, TESTOSTERONE
(GILT)

Speaking of hormones, let's take a moment to briefly discuss the major players. Without a doubt, the four most important hormones you must get in control are human growth hormone (Paul), testosterone (George), leptin (John), and in-sulin (Ringo).[3] The harmony that these four create together should be beautiful music. This harmonious invasion is the number one factor when considering fast, efficient fat loss, increased libido, and ripped, toned muscle. It doesn't stop there, either. When these four hormones are naturally being produced in their most effective, efficient manner, the home-ostasis of overall health is so amazing, it damn near makes you bulletproof. You must get these hormones working at their best in order to walk, talk, and breathe in your best body, period.

Growth Hormone

GH, or human growth hormone, is often referred to as "the fitness hormone" because of its powerful ability to burn fat, all while building beautiful, lean muscle at the same time. It is also commonly known as "the fountain of youth" hormone. This is because science has clearly proven that the less GH we have in our bodies, the faster we age. In other words, increasing your natural GH is essential to slowing the aging process. It enhances the immune system, your metabolism, and increases healthy cell regeneration. This healthy cell regeneration improves nails, skin, and hair significantly, maximizing your beauty while burning loads of fat. It has been proven to give us better mental clarity and alertness. Stress reduction is a direct result of increasing GH as well. Who could ask for much more? Research has also shown that nothing burns fat off your body faster than combining increased testosterone

---

[3] My hormone reference to the Beatles is quite simple. Paul is the fountain of youth (GH) and continues to create new music even in his 70's. George pushed everything to the limit as his testosterone dictated. John was a talent we always wanted more of (leptin) and quite simply lost way too early. And Ringo, well, let's just say, while a little bit of Ringo goes a long way, too much Ringo (insulin) is bad news. Come on now, this is funny!

with increased GH. This is literally the one-two knockout punch for fat bellies, thighs, and butts. Lucky for you, there are several very specific ways to increase your GH naturally, and we cover every single one of them in our program!

As your growth hormone improves you must provide them with powerful proactive Branched Chain Amino Acids. The very best on the planet can be found here: waketheforkup.com/shop/biotrust-products/bcaa-matrix/.

Insulin

Insulin is the key hormone when deciding whether your body will store the food you eat as fat on your body, or whether you will utilize those same calories to build shapely muscle and burn fat. It literally is the key hormone for turning off your fat storing mechanisms. When you eat the wrong foods for YOUR body, your pancreas secretes insulin, forcing your body to store those calories as fat. Over time, as you continue to feed yourself the wrong way, your body only gets worse with this process, causing you to store even more fat. This is because the same amount of insulin your body previously needed to control these calories now becomes less efficient, or resistant, forcing your body to produce even more insulin. As you become insulin resistant, again, you become more and more obese, putting your body in a **dis**eased state. Internal inflammation, leaky gut syndrome, diabetes, heart disease, and even some cancers are the direct result of being insulin resistant. So, we must get your insulin under control, once and for all. In fact, this is the number one reason people get type II diabetes. They are insulin resistant. According to the big brains at Harvard, combining the right styles and doses of resistance (weights, bands, body weight) exercises with the proper cardio training can reduce one's risk of getting type II diabetes by nearly 60%. Naturally, eating the correct foods at the right times for your body is equally important. In fact, a new study from the Genesis Prevention Center at the University Hospital in South Manchester, England suggests that you may be able to reset your insulin sensitivity with just two days a week of low to no sugar. Lucky for you, I have all the necessary tricks and scientifically proven methods to get your insulin back on track for you.

> *Once you do this, say "bye-bye" to annoying cravings. Say so long to the added risks of heart disease, pancreatic cancer, and obesity. Arrivederci to the nasty fat you currently have renting space on your body.*

Without these seven hormones working in harmony, you will NEVER have ripped abs or tight glutes. NEVER, EVER! Again, this superhuman, fat-burning system is designed specifically to get these hormones working optimally in record time. So please do not fret. Let's learn more about the remaining super hormones.

My supplement to help control blood sugar levels and enhance optimal insulin is IC 5™: waketheforkup.com/shop/biotrust-products/ic-5/.

Leptin

Leptin, much like insulin, plays a very important role when determining how and why we eat the way we do. Discovered in 1996 by Jeffrey Friedman, he gave this new hormone the name leptin, originating from the greek word "leptos," meaning thin. This is because the idea behind optimal leptin production is this—once your body reaches a certain level of fat, the leptin in this fat is released via the arcuate nucleus of the hypothalamus, telling our bodies essentially to stop eating (in other words, telling us to stop eating so we can stay thin). Yet, much like insulin, too much processed food, simple sugars, or trans fatty acids quickly blocks the normal function of this hormone. Add poor sleep and stress and before you know it, you are leptin resistant. Leptin resistance leads to being over-weight, becoming insulin resistant, and excessive inflamma-tion. Excessive inflammation has been attributed to many diseases and disorders, such as heart disease, diabetes, and cancer, as previously stated.

This is very important for two primary reasons. One is the fact that by the time you have become obese, your body is al-ready leptin resistant. This means that while you have plenty of leptin, your body is no longer able to recognize this, and therefore doesn't signal to your brain that you are satisfied (satiated), even when you do not need more food.

> *Secondly, if you are leptin resistant, chances are you are insulin resistant as well and now have double trouble.*

So, in addition to the excessive weight, you are now subject to injuring your pancreas, platelets, liver, and your heart, with diabetes knocking on your door.

As if this isn't bad enough, leptin sensitivity has also been shown to be directly connected to increased cortisol. This cat-abolic hormone eats away at our lean, toned muscle, while storing more body fat in our belly. So, it is very urgent that you begin to get this hormone working for you instead of against you as soon as possible. This is easily done in three ways. First, we need to replace foods that are *inflammatory promoting* (these are foods that contain chemicals called prostaglandins), such as cereals, prepackaged granola bars, and "healthy muffins" with healthy *anti-inflammation foods* such as spinach, cauliflower, wild fish, and walnuts. Second, we need to practice a healthy exercise plan that maximizes results in a minimum amount of time to keep cortisol in check. Lastly, we need to practice some form of stress management. Your program addresses all of these, precisely, in the correct manner.

Naturally, as you get this hormone functioning properly for you, you begin to stop the hunger pains and cravings. However, there is just one problem.

> *Theoretically, as you begin to burn more fat, eventually your body produces less than the optimal amount of leptin, and before you know it, maintaining the new fat loss becomes more and more difficult. This is often attributed as one of the number one reasons why it is much easier to burn the first 10 plus pounds of fat off your body, but it's so difficult to get rid of those last 5 to 10 pounds. This is why your Taste of Life; An Intellectual Eating Plan™ eating program will require one day of "super leptin loading" per week to ensure you control the cravings and burn off those last 5 to 10 pounds of fat, once and for all.*

More to come on this, specifically, in the nutrition section.

One side note of importance. It was recently discovered that while insulin resistance and leptin resistance share the same signaling pathways, and both occur in obese patients, obese men have higher insulin resistance, whereas obese women have more leptin resistance. This is why there will be slight differences for women with this program versus men. Specifically, as women get closer and closer to their ideal body fat levels, we will allow, in fact we encourage, them to have more than one "super leptin loading" day a week. More of this in the nutrition section to come. That's right ladies, you actually need more uploading than men do. How do you like them apples? ;-)

My supplement to help enhance optimal leptin levels is LeptiBurn™: waketheforkup.com/shop/biotrust-products/leptiburn/.

Your "Wake the Fork Up" Call
Testosterone

Testosterone is a word that often brings to mind images of hairy men, big trucks, and gladiator-style football. After all, testosterone is considered to be the principal male hormone, playing an important role in the development and maintenance of typical masculine characteristics, such as facial hair, muscle mass, and a deeper voice. So, why would women want healthy natural levels of testosterone? According to much research and an article written entitled "Women and Testosterone: An Interview with a Mayo Clinic specialist," the fact is, women produce it too, and it has more positive influences than you might think. So what does testosterone do for ladies? According to Paul Carpenter, M.D. from the Mayo Clinic, plenty good. Studies show that it helps maintain muscle, bone, and contributes to sex drive, or libido. There are also quality-of-life issues such as burning unwanted body fat in those often "lady associated" troubled zones, such as the buttocks, hips, and thighs, just to name a few. Increased natural testosterone is also beneficial to women's hearts and blood flow according to Harvard Medical School. It widens coronary arteries and increases red blood cells. Realize also, that a female body produces up to 40 times less testosterone than males, so do not worry, as you will not get "manly muscles" on this program as a result of **DIRT**™ improving your natural testosterone production. Instead, you will get increased energy, libido, and toned muscle, all while incinerating unwanted body fat and cellulite. And remember ladies, muscle takes up one-third of the space as fat.

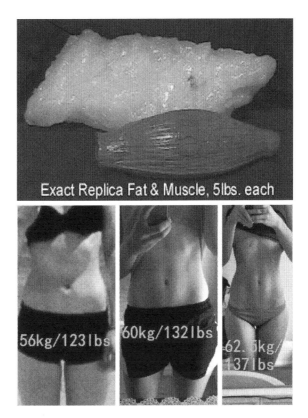

Exact Replica Fat & Muscle, 5lbs. each

56kg/123lbs 60kg/132lbs 62.5kg/137lbs

Notice how the pictures with more muscle, but heavier on the scale, look so much better and smaller? My point exactly!

Testosterone is also a very key component for men as well. From lean muscle to better sex, restful sleep, super strength, high energy, and fat burning, the list goes on and on. The trouble is, men's testosterone is dropping faster today than at any other time in history. This has directly impacted men as young as 20. The results? Fat, overstressed young men slowly becoming less and less interested in engaging their partners in a healthy, vital sex life. As you can imagine, this causes problems in all areas of their lives when testosterone is not functioning optimally. But, this does not need to be the case, even for men in their 30's, 40's, 50's and well beyond. In fact, a recent new study out of Australia has shown that it is lifestyle choices and NOT age that drops testosterone. This same study suggests that men in their 40's all the way up to their 70's should have healthy, natural levels of testosterone when practicing the right lifestyle choices. The adage, "it's a direct result of old age," turns out to be bogus yet again.

My supplement to help enhance optimal testosterone via increasing protein synthesis is Biotrust™ Low Carb Protein: waketheforkup.com/shop/biotrust-products/biotrust-low-carb/.

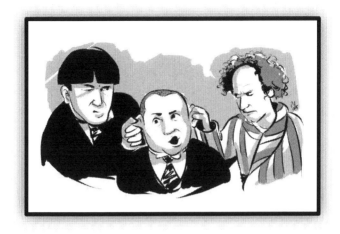

The Three Stooges
Estrogen, Cortisol, Ghrelin

Estrogen

Conversely to testosterone, most women, yet very few men, naturally produce higher levels of estrogen. Although unfortunately, due to poor nutrition, some men do experience higher levels. A high level of estrogen in men can cause man boobs, as well as fat storage in their derrière (ass), hips, and thighs (the pear shaped man with man boobs—yikes). While this condition may have made Kramer and George Costanza's father, from the famous sitcom *Seinfeld,* happy, so they could sell their "Bro" or "Manziere" (bras for men), most men find this uncomfortable at best. Guess what, so does your partner, whether they share it with you or not. Too much estrogen strips a man of testosterone as well. This phenomenon seriously begins to emasculate men. Don't let this happen, unless you are seriously thinking about a Chastity Bono to Chaz Bono transformation in reverse. Hey, I am not judging one bit, so get off your politically correct bully pulpit. But if you are here to get ripped abs and a Greek god bod, the old estrogen conversion is bad news.

And while healthy levels of estrogen can be good for a woman's overall health, too much estrogen is absolutely one of the main reasons why over 90 percent of my female clients, over the last 20 years, have come to me with a mission of losing excess fat in their hips, butt, and thighs.

Not to mention, many meats that have been pumped with estrogen, to help make them more "appealing to the manufacturers' bottom line profits" and get them to the market faster, increase estrogen. Add to this the low quality soy products sold to the masses (especially marketed to women), and many other estrogen mimicking foods and additives. The results are that many have more estrogen than desired (including women). I am not talking about a woman's *natural, healthy production* of estrogen. I am talking about unnecessary estrogen. I will discuss this topic more in the nutrition section, but I wanted to mention it, as many of you may have more estrogen than desired. Even worse, the more fat men and women have on their bodies, the more estrogen their body's produce due to an enzyme called aromatase. This enzyme actually converts healthy testosterone into unhealthy estrogen. Not good at all, my friends.

Now, while science has not proven that we can lower the *natural levels* of estrogen production in the body without taking prescribed medications (nor would we want to in women), the good news is that we can increase our natural hormonal secretion of testosterone to counterbalance this, as previously stated. We can also naturally begin to avoid estrogen mimicking foods and start melting away lots of that annoying fat storage in our butt, hips, and thighs.

As your body begins to cleanse itself of all the estrogenic chemicals, you will need to reduce GI inflammation and help improve intestinal health. Pro-X10™ is the best supplement for that: waketheforkup.com/shop/biotrust-products/pro-x10/.

Cortisol

Cortisol is another hormone often out of balance that causes a major increase in fat storage as well as many other ill effects. This hormone is often caused by stress, lack of sleep, and people that overwork themselves in their jobs, sports, workouts (you know, the human hamsters you see every day at the gym or in the parks running or doing endless cardio hour after hour at low to moderate intensities, week after week, month after month, with little to no results).

> *It turns out that this hormone is largely responsible for producing lots of fat, and often in the belly, even for those "who exercise regularly," albeit the wrong way.*

Go check out a marathon in your local area someday, and you will be amazed at how many runners out there are carrying way too much body fat. I, of course, am not talking about the elite runners who are literally pushing their bodies at eighty plus percentage max, most of the race. I am talking about the **L**ow **I**ntensity **T**raining herd (**LIT**), who grazily (a word I made up meaning slowly—like "cow grazing" slow) finish the race hours after the winners with upwards of 30% plus body fat. They are able to run a marathon, but still look like s*&t with their clothes off. Come on now, as that is as ineffective as it gets, in my opinion. You wanna run a marathon once in your life, as a sense of accomplishment, then go for it. Yet, if you aren't an elite runner with sub-three-hour times, forget about it as a viable fat-burning program. Not only will you not be receiving the best results with respect to time spent, but you could suffer from many overtraining injuries, including scar tissue on your heart. But enough about marathons.

Ah yes, the belly has been the biggest trouble area for men for centuries, although many women are now beginning to have their share of belly fat as a result of increased stress, over-training, sleep deprivation, and an increase in work-related responsibilities (not to mention, eating and training incorrectly). Even worse, as cortisol increases, protein synthesis (your ability to have lean, toned muscle) decreases and protein catabolism (a breakdown or re-duction in healthy lean muscle) increases, which eats away at our valuable muscle. The end result is a lower metabolic rate and even more belly fat getting stored. Until you gain control over your cortisol levels, you will never see your six pack abs.

Now don't get me wrong, cortisol is a natural hormone that our body produces in our adrenal glands that can make us stronger and burn fat in **short bursts**. But when this hor-mone starts to go into overdrive, it wreaks all kinds of havoc on our health quest. Probably the most profound result of too much cortisol is the catabolic response of breaking down lean, healthy muscle while adding bad fat, specifically on our waist-line. Belly fat is not only unattractive, it is linked to serious diseases and disorders in our body. The less lean muscle one has on their bodies, the more fat they will have. This is a "no-no" if you are looking to burn fat fast. In addition, scientists at the University of California found that cravings for un-healthy junk foods increased dramatically as a direct result of too much cortisol. This phenomenon will sabotage your jour-ney, and make you utilize your other hormones like insulin improperly as well. Many believe this is why exercising for long extended periods can be very bad for our bodies over time.

> *This may also be why those people that practice LIT (low intensity training) for long periods tend to binge eat more than most. We all know those people who train like lab rats for hours on end, week after week, month after month, only to show very little body composition/recompo-sition changes.*

In other words, you must learn to control your cortisol, once and for all.

Your **DIRT**™ program will help solve this problem with a few simple changes. You see, cortisol's number one nemesis is growth hormone (GH). The more GH our bodies are naturally producing, the more we are able to combat that nasty cortisol and burn that annoying belly fat.

> *To maximize your body's natural growth hor-mone secretion, you need to create more lactic acid in your workouts. The more lactic acid your body produces, the more GH your body must produce. You must also take short rest in-tervals in between your workout sets, and you must not train for hours on end. For all of the **DIRT**™ protocols, you rarely sit. Additionally, you must always fuse your lower body muscles with all of your movements. This gives you*

even more growth hormone production. Add some nice, restful sleep and you are well on your way. The result is, of course, Bye-Bye Belly Fat!

Take this natural supplement to help burn even more belly fat—BellyTrim™: waketheforkup.com/shop/biotrust-products/bellytrim-xp/.

Ghrelin

Ghrelin was discovered in 1999. It is often referred to as the "hunger hormone," as it was determined that this hormone more or less tells the brain when it is time to eat (stimulates hunger). In fact, when folks were injected with ghrelin, they ate on average 30% more than their study peers. Not only does ghrelin stimulate the hunger mechanism, it unfortunately slows metabolism and increases the body's ability to store unwanted fat, particularly in the abdominal region.

Even more troubling, common stressors, such as a lack of sleep, increase ghrelin, while lowering leptin. When this happens, it is noted that people will inadvertently choose foods higher in calories, processed sugar, and trans fats such as chocolate cake over a healthy and lean, wild salmon salad that is loaded with healthy walnuts and fat-burning vegetables.

You can guess the end result by now. Increased eating of bad foods and a massive increase in stored white adipose tissue WAT (the bad fat on your belly, buns, and legs) starts accumulating. Do not worry, however; our training and eating style gets your ghrelin under control in the most efficient way possible.

Garginia Cambogia has shown some great results with helping to tame ghrelin as well. Get the best right here: waketheforkup.com/shop/stevia-products/stur-liquid-garcinia-cambogia-for-appetite-control/.

Your "Wake the Fork Up" Call

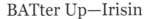

One "Super Cool" new hormone just recently discovered!

BATter Up—Irisin

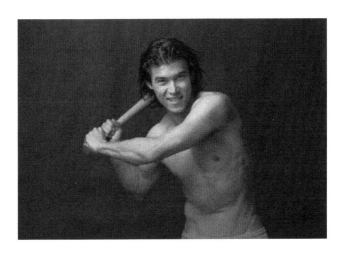

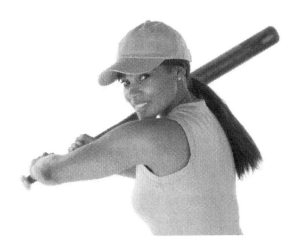

Those folks from Harvard Medical School never cease to amaze me. Some of their most recent research discovered a new hormone called IRISIN. Irisin literally speeds up your metabolism by increasing insulin sensitivity (remember, insulin sensitivity good -> insulin resistance bad). Even more amazing is the fact that irisin changes your white fat into brown fat! You see, it was once thought that adults only had a very limited amount of the good, metabolically active Brown Adipose Tissue (BAT) left over from childhood. This is the fat we want and need on our bodies to help reduce the white adipose tissue that chronically troubles the belly, hips, and thighs. Up until this discovery in 2012, it was thought that the majority of our BAT (good fat) was lost after infancy for good. (Ever wonder why 99% of all babies are chubby as hell and then suddenly, Boom, the fat all disappears? This is because the majority of their fat is BAT). In other words, we want more BAT (good, metabolically active fat) on

our bodies to burn the WAT (bad, disease-ridden fat) off of our bodies.

Brown fat cells don't store fat; they burn fat. "If your goal is to lose weight, you want to increase the number of brown fat cells and decrease your white fat cells," says Dr. Komaroff, a professor at Harvard Medical School. "Irisin does that. And those newly created brown fat cells keep burning calories post exercise." You know how we do this? We exercise in precisely the correct manner. When we do this, we can actually change bad fat into good fat. This is over the top, awesome people! We also know that much adult BAT likes to sit in the neck, upper back, and upper chest regions of the body. There is one simple trick to activate this fat burning BAT up to 300% more for you. Simply utilize ice therapy directly to this region of the body to help activate BAT—your good fat that helps to burn unwanted fat. This ice pack works best for rapid fat loss: waketheforkup.com/shop/amazon-products/core534/**.**

Are you beginning to understand why YOU must have a complete program that scientifically addresses and approaches things differently? A program that gets these powerful, proactive hormones working for you like they did when you were youthful and overflowing with energy? Why waste your hard-earned time, money, effort, and desire any longer? The solution is much easier than people make it out to be, but it's not so simple even a caveman can accomplish it.

The truth almost always lies somewhere in between. The truth to six pack abs and a tight sexy booty style of training is about to be revealed, once and for all. Simply shoot here for instant access: waketheforkup.com/programs/.

Listen up gang, I know that on any given day of the week, you can find literally hundreds of different fitness programs and diet protocols. However, if you want to get these super, fat fighting, lean muscle building hormones working their very best for you, in the shortest amount of time, you must do **Dynamic Integrated Results-based Training™ (DIRT™).** The secret is in the proprietary combination of the three most effective styles of training put together in a perfect hybrid format.

The first workout strategically manipulates your lactic acid production and is called DIRT™ Focused Form Hypertrophy/ Time Under Tension Training. With very simple, yet specific changes, we can guarantee maximum results without suffering from common over-training injuries. The second strategy integrates a very effective metabolic conditioning training style. It is called the DIRT™ Body Watts Meta-Blast. This is not simply circuit training. The simple, yet particular details of this style specifically trigger metabolic training much faster and efficiently than normal circuit training. The third style you will incorporate is the DIRT™ Explosive Strength Training Plus program. Different from other "normal" strength training programs, we make a few simple, yet specific changes that drastically impact your results in record time, as the devil is in the details. Don't be fooled. The synergistic

*properties involved with these patented train-
ing programs ensure your body releases all the
great hormones it is currently neglecting to
produce more of, all while slowing down the release of the evil fat-promoting hormones.*

Remember, it is the three programs being used in the exact prescribed manner that guarantees your success with all of the troubled fat zones. And while many of you may be interested in only doing one of the **DIRT**™ training formats, the reality is that most of you have undesirable fat storage in more than one of these trouble areas. The fact of the matter is that every one of the **DIRT**™ programs increases all of your super hormones, while decreasing your fat storage hormones. Even more importantly, if you **only** do one style of this workout system, you will inevitably hit a nasty plateau, as your body adapts to the one style of exercise. Not to mention, you are likely to be susceptible to becoming another statistic of overtraining and injuries, which will, no doubt, sabotage your fatburning goals. So, get the notion of only using one format out of your head now. Got it? Good!

Please understand that I am not saying that there are specific *exercises* that can *spot reduce fat*. That is to say, crunches will not reduce fat in your stomach any more than hip extensions (butt extensions) will blast fat from your ass. This concept is called spot reduction and is not possible, *for the most part* (see Fat Fader below). I repeat, I did not do hundreds upon hundreds of abdominal exercises to get awesome abs. Believe it or not, people still ask me and my clients this often. Many are amazed that the majority of our workout time does not even involve direct isolation abdominal exercises. I will say this again; I do not do hundreds of abdominal exercises to achieve my ripped abs, and neither should you. This is because specific exercises strengthen, tone, and shape certain muscles. They do not, however, burn fat from that specific spot or area. I am not saying this and want to make myself clear.

I AM, HOWEVER, SAYING THAT MUCH SCIENTIFIC RESEARCH HAS PROVEN THAT THERE ARE SPECIFIC **EXERCISE STYLES** THAT MAXIMIZE FAT LOSS. AND, EVEN BETTER, FAT LOSS IN OUR SPECIFIC TROUBLED ZONES! THIS IS PRECISELY WHAT THIS NEW FANTAS-TIC METHOD OF EXERCISE IS ALL ABOUT. This is EX-ACTLY WHAT *DYNAMIC INTEGRATED RESULTS-BASED TRAINING*™ DOES FOR YOU! Exercise Science has come a long way folks, and you are about to benefit like you never have before.

Even more so, if I can get you to train in a fasted state (on an empty stomach), your body will literally activate cyclic AMP and AMP kinases, forcing the breakdown of fat and gly-cogen for energy, instead of lean muscle mass. The Swedish School of Sport and Health Sciences has shown that exercising in a fasted state helps burn calories more efficiently, while in-creasing muscle oxidative potential. The primary reason for this was increasing mitochondrial biogenesis. According to fitness expert Ori Hofmekler, author of *The Warrior Diet,* you can literally redesign your physique as a direct result of this mitochondrial biogenesis.

> *What is so exciting about this is the fact that your body actually preserves and protects your active muscle from wasting itself. In other words, exercising first thing in the morning on an empty stomach absolutely burns much more fat, while preserving much needed lean muscle. Now, don't panic if you are unable to work out on an empty stomach. There are more than*

*enough great benefits in this programming to
get you to where you want to be in record time.
Doing it on an empty stomach will simply get
you there faster.*

In addition, and perhaps even more exciting, I have discovered a topical product that has offered tremendous fat loss
in the areas to which it was applied. I have used the product
myself for some time now, and I can 100% say that the area I
applied the topical gel to lost more than three times as much
body fat than the untreated area. The reason for this, again,
is that science keeps getting better and better, and they have
found a proprietary blend of the right stuff that ACTUALLY
makes this happen. The key ingredient that has the most profound impact on these specific troubled zones is called AMI-
NOPHYLLINE. I have tested many of these products over the
years and, unbeknownst to me, this was the key ingredient responsible for real fat reduction.

*This was first brought to my attention by none
other than Tim Ferris from* The Four Hour
Body. *As Tim puts it, "In plain* **Ingrish,** *for
decades, the consensus among exercise professionals has been that spot reduction—reducing
fat in one specific body area—is impossible, a
myth." He continues, "I long assumed this was
the case until I asked the hypothetical question:
if we assume there might be an effective mechanism for spot reduction, what would it look
like? It seemed that one answer would be a topical lotion that inhibits the A-2 receptor or
blocks phosphodiesterase." Topical lotions that
contain the correct amount of aminophylline
do this. That is to say, when appropriately pre-*

scribed exercise and intellectual eating are present, rubbing this cream in your troubled zones would, in fact, encourage your body to burn fat say, off your ass or abs, quicker and more efficiently than in your face, for example. This is very important, as we all have trouble fat deposit areas where we need to rid the fat faster. Voila, spot reduction, with proper training and eating, can happen!

What is the name of the product you ask? Wait for it...***Fat Fader***. Tim uses a similar product called Celluthin, and while it and Acavar both worked, only **Fat Fader** worked for me without irritating my skin. It is literally half the price of the other products, as well. Believe me, it is not like the other 99% of those products being sold for fat loss. This one actually works. You can go right here to order your supply today: waketheforkup.com/shop/fat-fader/.

Remember, all the science and research has already been done for you and the programming absolutely works. To make it fail proof for you, I have designed a workout manual for you. Full photo descriptions of exactly what to do, how to do it and when. But there's more. Because so many have expressed an interest in being able to work along with me while training, I have designed 12 **DIRT**™ exercise videos just for YOU. These are 12 totally different workouts based on the scientific methodologies that have been proven to get you results fast. **Dynamic Integrated Results-Based Training**™ is literally one of the most advanced fat-burning exercise systems available. The research and results are groundbreaking with this total body transformation system. This is the only place on the planet you can get it—waketheforkup.com/programs/.

CHAPTER EIGHT
Cardio that Rocks—"Moves Like Jagger"

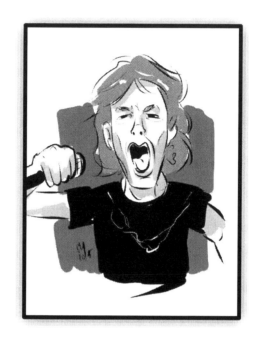

"Anything worth doing is worth overdoing."

—*Mick Jagger*

Bittersweet

Summer 2011, Chicago Speedway, Joliet, Illinois

Today is the day. Finally, I was able to get one of my all-star clients, Brian Darflinger, to trust me and try out his new cardio formula in a fashion that he could appreciate. Let me rewind. Two years prior, a client had approached me, wanting to better his overall body composition, as he had been competing in triathlons for several years now, but didn't feel like he was getting the best results for the time he was committing. He had initially received some positive results in his overall physical appearance and fitness level, but as time went on, he just couldn't seem to lose that last bit of fat in his abs and love handles (oblique area). As I began to explain to him the trouble with Low Intensity Training (LIT), combined with no significant resistance training, he reluctantly started to listen. You see, many marathon runners and triathletes carry more body fat than they want and need. This is predominantly because they are limiting their good hormones, maximizing their bad hormones, and literally burning lean muscle tissue instead of fat. They also often suffer from overuse training injuries and aches. Not to mention, unless they are one of the "elite triathletes," they rarely test their aerobic and anaerobic thresholds and, therefore, their bodies quickly adapt to this extended long-term cardio routine. The results equal increased cortisol and ghrelin, along with decreased growth hormone and testosterone. They also begin to suffer from the dreaded injury cycle that often accompanies this type of training. Furthermore, they carry more fat than many, even though they are actually quite fit.

Again, Darfman was a little suspicious, but he decided to trust me and began to slowly start training with my **DIRT**™ system. The trouble was that guys like this love to compete. So, I had to create a way he could compete in races, and yet not do it for these, oftentimes, damaging overextended triathlon bouts. So, I decided to invite him to compete with me and some friends in a race called *The Warrior Dash*. This is a rough and tough obstacle course that challenges both your endurance and strength systems much like **DIRT**™ does. It is only a distance of 5k, and therefore would be considerably less time/distance than his usual triathlons. As the race began, I ran alongside of him for approximately the first third of the race course. But then, the competitor in me came out and I bid him adieu and started to leave him behind. In a short period of time, I pulled away from him substantially, and as I glanced back, I could not see him in the crowd. I was confident he would finish, but was fearing he had not been pushing his anaerobic and aerobic thresholds, as we had discussed, and would therefore simply fall into the steady state rate he had grown accustomed to with his triathlon training. I thought to myself, 'This will be a good lesson to reinforce why he must be diligent with my **DIRT**™ training formula,' as he is a very competitive guy and would not be happy getting smoked by me in the race. So I pushed on, and by the time I hit the Cargo Net Wall Climb, my system was beginning to get a little taxed. When I got to the top of the wall, I looked back, and again did not see the Darfman. I climbed down the cargo wall and kept trucking forward.

With less than three minutes left in the race, we were hit with a dozen hills...up and down, up and down. This time, when I looked back, however, the Darfman suddenly seemed to pop into my view out of nowhere. 'WTH!' I thought. Where the heck did he come from? I was not worried, as he was still a good 20 yards behind me. Next came the Fire Leap, and as I jumped over it, I decided not to look back this time. After all, now my competitive juices were flowing, and there was no way in hell I was gonna let the coach (me) lose the race. This brought me to the last obstacle, which was the dreaded mud crawl under barbed wire. As I entered the pit filled with water and mud, I realized I needed to dunk my head under in order to safely be below the barbed wire. As I first came up for air, I could barely see even one foot in front of me as a direct result of literally having mud in my eyes! 'Forget about it,' I thought, as I rushed under this wire like Blind Melon Chitlin.

As I climbed out of the pit and ran to the finish line, I crossed with a confidence of both pride and satisfaction. Not only had I won the race (or so I thought), but my student obviously had been practicing my training protocol, as his strong finish had indicated. Seconds later, I rushed straight to the watering hole to wash the mud off my body and out of my eyes, and I still literally could not see clearly for minutes, until after multiple rinses. The finish line was mass hysteria, as competitors were trying to rinse mud out of every orifice for 10 minutes at a time. I had lost all of my friends, as they were all blinded at the finish line as well.

Fifteen minutes later, I found Darfman. I congratulated him and said, "Man, I was really proud and surprised to see you catching up with me at the end there. I almost thought you were going to beat me." The look in his muddy eyes told me all I needed to know, and I simply said, "No way, dude!" He started laughing and said, "Yep! I passed you in the mud trench, brother. I couldn't see for sure, but I think I beat you!" Sure enough, as we would find out the next day when our times were posted, he beat me by 1.3 seconds. That was a bittersweet moment where the student surpassed the coach.

So, when I asked him, "How in the world did you catch me?" he simply stated, "I used your 90-60-30 second training protocol." Unbelievable! I was beaten by my student, who was using my training method. He said, "Although I felt like I was gonna die with the level 10 push, I knew it was only for 30 seconds, so I literally started closing the gap on you every three minutes." I simply replied, "You must be a GOT Damm Genius, Gump!" (while I like profanity, I do not use God's name in vain), and smiled with feelings of pride. Not only had my plan worked, but when he took his muddy shirt off, the cat had lost over four inches on his waistline, something he had never accomplished before. He had gotten everything he had asked for and more...bragging rights by whipping the coach's butt in the race. And therefore, I changed the 90-60-30 to the **DIRT™y Darfman-Fat Blaster**. He still continues to race these shorter, more High Intensity Interval Style races, and dominates his age group. Rock on Darfman, Rock on!

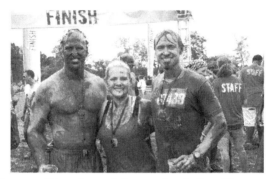

The Champ (Darfman) is on the left... He made me call
him that for one full year.

Cardio that Rocks!

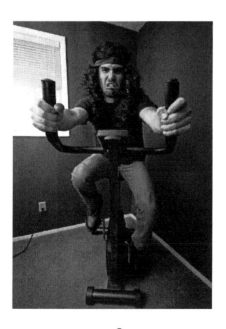

For your Cardio Routines, you may have already guessed that there are three different styles as well. All are designed specifically to maximize your results in the absolute shortest amount of time. And yes, ALL ARE DESIGNED TO PULVERIZE FAT LIKE A BUTCHER ON A PIG!

Sure, aerobic exercise of any kind will help you burn some calories. However, a significant number of studies show that long distance, long duration cardio training protocols with the usual *Low Intensity Training* style known as **LIT** do very little to enhance fat loss. LIT also has been proven to increase cortisol, decrease GH, and increase binge eating. In addition, some studies are now showing that extended cardio sessions can actually cause scar tissue to develop in our hearts and cardiovascular systems as well. In 2012, a report published in the *Mayo Clinic Proceedings* suggested that the damage endurance athletes do to their hearts actually adds up over time. Repeated long-distance racing can cause a buildup of scar tissue in the heart, which can lead to the development of patchy myocardial fibrosis in up to 12% of LIT participants. "It's a cumulative thing," said Dr. James O'Keefe, of the Mid-Atlantic Heart Institute.

> *In fact, most experts in body transformation consider LIT to be the absolute worst form of exercise you can do, period.*

Sure it will burn some calories while you are actually exercising, but it doesn't boost your metabolism after your workout. It doesn't increase testosterone and GH. It doesn't make you more insulin and/or leptin sensitive. In other words, it does NOT put your hormones in an optimum environment. I will say this again—the normal way most people train in a cardiovascular manner, with a long drawn out steady state rate of exercise, is probably the least efficient form of exercise there is. But of course that doesn't mean that our cardio days are completely over.

Let's face it, you can go weeks without food and days without water, if you absolutely must, in an emergency situation. But you can only survive on this planet without oxygen for a few minutes, in most cases, before you drop dead, guys and gals. And yes, our three resistance programs definitely get your oxygen transport (cardiovascular system) working better than any other style of resistance training. But, to remove cardio altogether would be very foolish, in my opinion. However, make no mistake about it, there is a much more effective way to perform cardiovascular conditioning without overtraining, reducing muscle, and making yourself susceptible to unnecessary injuries.

Conversely, **HIIT** stands for High Intensity Interval Training. This is a method of cardiovascular training that is becoming increasingly popular, as people are finally catching on to its amazing benefits. This technique allows you to throw very intense efforts or bursts of speed into your cardiovascular exercise of choice, along with some "recovery phases" as well, so you do not redline your body too quickly.

*This style of training is key for many specific reasons. One, this style of training has been scientifically proven to drastically increase EPOC or **Excess Post-exercise Oxygen Consumption** (informally called **after burn**).*

This is defined as a measurably increased rate of oxygen intake following strenuous activity. This creates the magic needed to transform your body, as it is literally connected to increased metabolism, increased growth hormone, increased thermogenesis, and an increase in your muscle ATP. The EPOC effect is obviously greatest a few hours after you complete your exercise, but one study from the *European Journal of Applied Physiology* showed that EPOC can have a powerful effect on our bodies even 38 hours post-workout.

Secondly, most people believe that any type of cardio is smart heart training. But again, this is only part of the story.

You see, most folks forget that we have three muscle fiber types—slow twitch (aerobic), fast twitch, and super fast twitch (anaerobic). And guess what? Our heart is made up of fast and super fast twitch fibers as well. So, all these years of only training your LIT style of cardio was only training half of your heart's muscle fibers at best (as your fast and super fast twitch make up roughly 50% of your heart muscle).

And believe me, if you aren't pushing yourself in a manner that challenges your anaerobic threshold with volume and velocity of movement, then you are not training your heart's anaerobic properties. Once you learn to integrate this system into your new routine, the synergistic biochemical response will have you increasing all the right hormones, while massively burning more fat.

Your "Wake the Fork Up" Call

New research has shown us that not only will slow steady rate cardio training (LIT) give us less fat burn for the day, but even worse that it can cause scar tissue to develop in our cardiac muscles! It only trains our slow twitch muscle fibers (not our fast twitch and super fast twitch). It throws our fat-burning, muscle-building hormones out of balance. Remember, that training over 45 minutes at any one given time will also deplete our body of the super fat-burning hormones we are looking for as well. The bottom line is that working out for hours on end at a slow steady rate is bad for our fat-burning quest, and it is one of the very reasons why we see so many overly fat people fail on those types of programs.

Realize that we all have a perceived rate of exertion. This is the level of effort we apply when moving our bodies to perform a function. I have put together a fun chart for you to use when estimating your level of exertion. So please do not get caught up in the speeds I am hypothetically suggesting. The important aspect is that YOU work at an appropriate level that allows YOUR body to hit the suggested perceived rates of exertion as shown on the scale. We all have different bodies with different levels of fitness, function, and health-related issues. Therefore, you will need to take some time to understand where your level is at this time. In other words, let's use this chart as an example for levels of exertion with your specific, chosen exercises. For example, if I suggest you warm up at a level 5, looking at the chart, you may walk at a brisk pace. This will change as you become more and more conditioned, so hang in there. You're Fat-Burning Machine is in there and is desperately trying, yearning, and begging you to unleash it! Bearing this in mind, let's take a look at the scale now:

Exertion Level	Activity Example
1	Sleeping
2	Sitting in a Chair Reading
3	Getting up out of that chair and walking to the kitchen or bathroom— shouldn't require a lot of energy ;)
4	Walking at a Slow Pace/Clip
5	Walking at a Brisk Pace/Clip
6	A Slow Jog, Bike Ride, Skate
7	Activity that Gets You Out of Breath—You Can Talk, but your Breathing is Labored
8	You No Longer Want to Talk, because the Energy Level Required is Taking your Full Concentration! It's Hard!
9	You are Pushing at a Level that Will No Longer Allow You to Carry on a Conversation and You Will Not Talk—You're Moving Baby!
10	All-Out Exertion—A Bear is Chasing You, and You are Running for your Life! Get Moving!!!

My three **DIRT**™**y** HIIT cardio routines are a combination of the very best protocols to guarantee maximum results in a minimum amount of time. How little, you ask? Many folks get great results in as little as nine minutes a day, two to three days a week. No one ever does more than three days a week and never longer than 39 minutes a session. I'll teach you exactly what to do and at exactly the precise exertion level (intensity level). Better yet, I have designed three cardio videos for you that allow you to train anywhere with absolutely zero equipment required. No gym memberships needed and no spending thousands of dollars on cardio equipment.

DIRT™**y** cardio is some of the most effective, powerful exercises on the planet and you can only get it right here: waketheforkup.com/programs/.

Part Three

CHAPTER NINE

Your <u>Primary</u> <u>M</u>ethod of <u>E</u>ating & the Power of Three

"One man's food is another man's poison."

—*Lucretius (99 B.C. - 55 B.C.)*

Your Primary M.E. and the Power of Three™ for Nutrition consists of three basic principles. **One**, you first must learn what YOUR Nutritional Metabolic Type is. After all, one man's food is another man's poison. The "one-size-fits-all" protocol that so many other "health experts" push simply will not work for everyone. For example, if you have a Carbohydrate Nutritional Metabolic type, you only need to fuel one to two times a day, whereas Protein Metabolic types need to eat three to four times daily. **Two**, you MUST learn the secret power of Intelligent Eating, as I like to call it. This powerful, well-researched approach will literally have you feeling superhuman in record time. Why? Because it is the only style of eating that optimizes your Seven Super Fat-Burning Hormones. **Three**, you will learn to navigate clear of those foods that are absolute poison for your nutritional metabolic type and sabotage your fat-burning goals, once and for all. These **three simple steps** will have you on your way to fitness stardom in no time. The synergy of all three is the magic potion. It will literally burn fat off your body faster than any other nutrition plan available, period. Even better, the foods are delicious and nutritious. But before I dig right into the metabolic typing, I would like to share a few wake-up moments with you.

By now, I feel you can guess that my nutrition plan will be like nothing you have seen before in most ways, and a little like others in a few ways. However, the combination of which is unique and completely opposite of what many so-called professionals have been trying to force-feed you, in their ongoing attempts to "dumb things down" for the masses. Along these very lines, I will also discuss the ever so popular and ever so profitable food industry engine that cleverly and scientifically creates, processes, markets, and sells food for one reason and one reason only—maximum profits, period. Included in this will be a brief mention of big pharmaceutical companies, along with the AMA and all the medicines they are force "feeding" you, in hopes that you will choose their route instead of learning how to nourish your body healthfully, once and for all. Not to mention the massive amounts of "diet" and "weight loss" products, foods, pills, and drinks that you are bombarded with on a daily, hour to hour, and minute to minute basis. Combine this with the daily stresses, schedules, and lack of good understanding, and it is no wonder that we are the leading overweight, undernourished (I will explain this later), and overmedicated country in the world today. The very thought of all of these forces coming together and working against you is enough to make me nauseous.

However, please know that the bulk of my conversation will be on teaching you how to eat right for **YOUR nutritional metabolic type**, in **YOUR proper intellectual eating window** formula. The research has an accumulated history of over 80 years and counting, and it is some of the most amazing, unique, and truly beneficial nutrition research available. Even more exciting, some of the research is cutting-edge information that is less than five years old (as of the publication of this book). Yet, it is presented in an easy to understand and easy to implement format. It will enable you, once and for all, to properly nourish your body with the right amounts, types, and combinations of foods to guarantee that you continue to succeed in your quest to become the leanest, healthiest fat-burning machine out there. It will teach you to identify and create your Primary Method of Eating in a simple three-step process through my patented *Primary M.E. and the Power of Three™ Programming.* Much like your exercise and lifestyle coaching programs, three simple, effective steps are really all it takes. Stick with the program, and in no time you will be burning fat more effectively than a chef roasting a pig on a spitfire. But before you can do this, you must first decide right here, right now, that you will read, not skim, this entire portion of the book. It is the only way you will succeed at continuing to master your fat-burning quest. Are you up for the challenge? Are you ready to embrace the new you? I know that your answer is yes. I know you are going to become one of my WTFU Warriors, a leader in your home, community, and group. Therefore, I feel it is time that YOU become informed. It is time that YOU take responsibility and become a leader in your nutritional choices and awareness. It is time for YOU to **Wake The Fork Up®**!

Your "Wake the Fork Up" Call
The Food Industry is a Business

The Food Industry (those companies who sell us food, i.e., agriculture, big food companies, grocery stores, restaurants, etc.) are in business to make money, first and foremost. In order to do this, they must encourage us to eat their food as opposed to others. It is a simple business bottom line, if you really step into your common sense corner and think about it.

Consequently, many of these companies sacrifice vital nutritious systems and safety guidelines in order to sell more food. Naturally, they have studied your habits, likes, and dislikes; they have tried to make food as flavorful, convenient, and readily available as possible. Virtually every corner, in any major town or city, has some form of food available, whether it be through a grocery store, restaurant, convenience mart, gas station, or even a liquor store. The choices today are endless, and the opportunity to over-consume is lurking around every corner. While most of this may sound somewhat familiar to you, perhaps my next statement will not. Did you know that many high-level food industry executives are in a relentless pursuit to find scientifically proven ways to make you eat more? THAT'S RIGHT, EXECUTIVES EARNING MILLIONS OF DOLLARS A YEAR WITH ONE PURPOSE IN MIND... GETTING YOU TO CONSUME MORE OF THEIR PRODUCT! It's absolutely true. They could care less about your health and wellness, despite the fact that the world is in a major crisis regarding obese individuals and all of the **dis**eases and **dis**orders directly related to poor nourishment. Yes, malnourishment. Contrary to popular belief, one does not need to be starving in a Third World country to be malnourished. In fact, here in America, most overweight, overly fat individuals suffer from malnutrition. They are literally starving for the right kinds of foods and vital nutrients. This is a fact, my friends. Wake up!

But these titans of the food industry are not concerned with malnutrition, as I have described it. Their primary concern is to get you to eat as much of their "designed foods" as they can.

In fact, according to Dr. David Kessler, "Higher sugar, unhealthy fats, and salt make you want

128

to eat more, and the food industry not only knows this; they count on it."

When Dr. Kessler (2009) interviewed an executive in the food industry who he called the equivalent of "Henry Ford" of mass produced food, he was amazed at how well these execs knew exactly how to make you eat more and more. To protect his business, the food exec did not want to be identified, but he was remarkably candid when discussing his company's approach.

> *"The food industry creates dishes to hit the three points of the compass: sugar, fat, and salt." This combination makes the food compelling, indulgent, and even hedonic, which ultimately gives you pleasure and makes you want to eat more.*

When Dr. Kessler asked a restaurant food consultant to describe the three points of said compass contained in some foods commonly found in popular restaurants today, here were some of his results.

> *Potato skins: Typically the potato is hollowed out, and the skin is fried, which provides a substantial surface area for what he calls "fat pickup." Then some combination of bacon bits, sour cream, and cheese is added. Not to mention, the potato itself turns to sugar quickly in the body. Add a sugary drink to this, and you are left with fat on fat on fat on fat. To make matters worse, this dish is also loaded with salt and sugar.*

> *Buffalo wings: Start with the fatty parts of a chicken, which get deep fried. Then they're served with creamy*

or sweet dipping sauce that's heavily salted. Usually, they're par-fried at a production plant, and then fried again at the restaurant, which essentially doubles the fat. That gives you sugar on salt on fat on fat on fat.

Spinach dip: The spinach provides little more than color and a bit of appeal; a high-fat, high-salt dairy product is the main ingredient. It's a tasty dish of salt on fat. Add a sugary drink to the mix, and you're look-ing to eat as much of it as they can put on the table.

Chicken tenders: They are so loaded with batter and fat that the consultant jokes that they are a UFO—an unidentified FRIED object. Additionally, there is salt and sugar along with said fat.

White Chocolate Mocha Frappuccino: Served at Star-bucks, this drink is comprised of coffee diluted with a mix of sugar, fat, and salt.

This list goes on and on and on. And they are damn good at their jobs. They can even take what seems to be the healthy choice on the menu and zap it into a "crave-able" food.

Example at hand, the Cheesecake Factory's Buffalo Blasts: Chicken breast, cheese, and spicy buffalo sauce, all stuffed in a spiced salty wrapper and fried until crisp. Served with celery sticks and blue cheese dressing. For a moment, the food con-sultant simply laughs. "What can I say? That's fat, sugar, and salt," he responds. The chicken breast allows you to suspend your reasoning and guilt, because it suggests a low-fat dish, and the celery sticks also hint at something healthy. But the cheese layer is at least 50 percent fat and carries a load of salt, and the buffalo sauce adds a layer of sugar on salt. The dough wrapper—a simple (sugary) carbohydrate—is fried and so absorbent that he called it a "fat bomb." As their conversation wound down, he walked Dr. Kessler to the door. Then with the certainty that only an insider could have, he simply stated, **"the food industry is a manipulator of the consumers' minds and desires"** (Kessler 2009, 18-20).

Other research showed many more detailed explanations as to how they can manipulate you to eat more and more. From *taste* to *texture, variety* to *concentration, and quantity* to *dynamic contrast,* the industry knows every angle.

> *In fact, some food industry leaders have become so "good" at their job that they have actually created foods that stimulate our opioid circuitry, which is the body's pleasure system. The "opioids," also known as endorphins, are chemicals produced in the brain that have rewarding effects similar to drugs such as morphine and heroin.*

Heroin and morphine, people! Stimulating the opioid circuitry with food drives us to eat more and more. The desire can become as strong as that of any drug addict looking for their next fix.

When Michele Foley, a food scientist at Frito Lay, was giving a talk called "Simply Irresistible—Understanding High Levels of Satisfaction and What it Means," her key research question was, "What are the attributes that increase craveability for products?" During this "seminar," Foley pointed out five key influences on irresistibility in order of importance: calories, flavor hits, ease of eating, meltdown, and early hit. **"Those are the attributes that drive cravings for you to eat," she said.** Within the framework of her five keys, she emphasized the power of cheese and other dairy flavors to contribute to irresistibility in nacho cheese Doritos. These Doritos have many sought-after attributes—multiple flavor hits from three different cheeses and various milks and creams with salt and oil adding to the pleasure. There's also a crunch and hardness with the first bite, followed by a meltdown that turns the chips into a sauce in the mouth.

> *The end result was this: Foley was clear about her business research. "It's not about predicting what consumers will like; it's about being sure," she said (Kessler 2009).*

Combine that with a multitude of mass marketing and carefully considered ambiance suggests that the food industry knows exactly what they are doing. They are finding more and more ways to make you eat over and over, regardless of the impact. Not to mention, the more you eat foods like this, the more your body and mind will actually crave these foods. This cycle is addictive, destructive, and can become all consuming. They are well aware of these factors, and yet they are the very ones who make claims in the mass market as to why their food is just fine, if not healthy for you.

> *Selling a cereal that rhymes with "Heerios" to lower your cholesterol, people? Give me a break! Soluble fiber is where this research originates, and "Heerios" is a poor source of fiber, calorie for calorie, at best!*

I will show just how poor in the pages to follow. This is only one little example of the total BS the mass media is selling us. It simply is not true, folks. You must become smarter than the average bear if you want to succeed in this arena. You must become a leader, and not a follower. Big business, government, and industry has done enough damage to our societies as a whole. Do not continue to allow this to happen to you.

CHAPTER TEN
The Bermuda Triangle of Foods

"The key to eating healthy is to avoid any food you see advertised on the television."

—Unknown

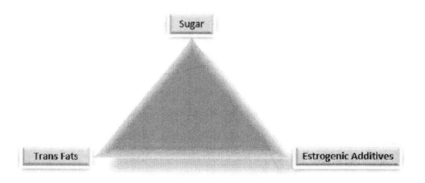

The Bermuda Triangle of Processed Foods

What would be the most damaging and addictive food out there? By far, I would have to say those processed foods (foods that come in a can, box, plastic bag, from a fast food restaurant, etc.) that contain the highest percentage of cautious carb sugars and toxic chemicals, such as trans fats and estrogenic producing chemicals.

Realize one simple fact; in order for these foods to sit on shelves day after day, month after month, and, for some, even year after year, the food industry must do ONE thing and one thing only. They must strip the foods they started with of vital nutrients, replacing them with harmful chemicals, preservatives, and various forms of sugar, PERIOD! How else could food sit on shelves for this amount of time and not spoil?

Sugars, chemicals, and trans fatty acids are the three biggest culprits. These things are slowly poisoning our society, and the food industry doesn't care one bit. The reason I say this is simply because every nutritional metabolic type can suffer dire consequences by over-consuming these products (even the Carbo Type).

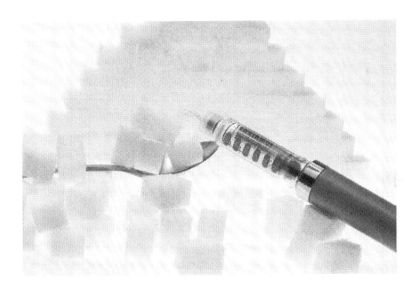

The Sugar Monsters

What are cautious carbs? Very simply, these are foods that break down into sugar very quickly in our bodies once we ingest them. Of course, sugar and all of its forms (fructose, sucrose, dextrose, high fructose corn syrup, etc.) enter the bloodstream with a very high blood sugar response. Yet many other foods enter with just as much damaging properties.

For example, did you know that a piece of white bread has a glycemic index of 100? This means that this bread enters our system as quickly as if you were drinking sugar water.

The consequences of such consumption forces our bodies to produce massive amounts of insulin that in turn stores most of these calories as fat on your body. And for protein metabolic types, this sugar stain is even worse. Other examples are most white flour-based products, juices, soft drinks, and sports drinks. White potatoes, pasta, and certainly bread can convert to fat on our bodies in a New York minute. Furthermore, most processed foods have a very negative effect on our bodies. And "pure natural sugar" can be one of the worst culprits. That's right folks, just because it is "natural" does not mean that it is good for everyone, especially at the excessive levels the average person consumes, oftentimes unknowingly. Just because it doesn't look like sugar or taste like sugar does not mean it is not sugar producing in our bodies. Sugar is literally hiding in every single processed food on the shelves, even if they do not show up on the label. This "added sugar" is everywhere, and it puts fat on our bodies in record time.

In addition, we now know that all of this sugar we are eating causes massive inflammation to the body internally. *This is what leading nutritionist Brenda Watson calls Silent inflammation.* She adds that it happens internally and often originates in the gut as a result of a leaky gut, or intestines that have become too permeable due to a poor diet, lack of gut-healing nutrients, stress, and other factors. Silent inflammation does not heal itself. You can't feel silent inflammation or see it. This silent inflammation is now thought to be one of the proximate, root causes to diseases such as diabetes, increased levels of triglycerides and LDL (bad cholesterol), increases in plaque and blockage of arteries or heart disease, and even some forms of cancer, such as breast and colon cancer, just to name a few. This is no joke folks. Outside of making your body very obese, becoming addicted to these Sugar Monsters can be downright deadly over time. I will say it again. In our bodies, inflammation is extremely damaging and over time, wreaks major havoc on our overall system.

Even worse, once we over-consume all these products filled with sugar, we actually begin to crave and want more of them like a drug addict wants more drugs. This is what I call the *Sugar Monsters! The Sugar Monsters are literally the number one reason why so many people fail at their nutrition and therefore end up overly fat and out of shape, with literally hundreds of damaging, yet connected side effects. To make matters worse, the food industry is well aware of this factor and works hard to hide and deny the facts, so you continue to overeat their food.*

Top 10 Sugar Monster Sources:

1) SODA-POP/SOFT DRINKS
2) FRUIT JUICES
3) SPORTS DRINKS, SUGARY TEAS, ENERGY DRINKS
4) FRAPPUCCINOS, LATTES OR WHATEVER ELSE YOU ARE CALLING COFFEE
5) CAKES, COOKIES, PIES, AND PASTRIES IN GENERAL
6) MOST ALL BREADS (Bagels) WITH THE EXCEPTION OF SPROUTED BREADS, SOME ANCIENT GRAIN BREADS & SOME GLUTEN FREE BREADS

7) MOST PROCESSED (BOXED, CANNED, OR PLASTIC WRAPPED) FOODS
8) CHIPS, PRETZELS, CRACKERS, CRISPS, CEREAL
9) NATURAL SUGAR, HIGH FRUCTOSE CORN SYRUP, SUCROSE, DEXTROSE, ETC.
10) SOME HIGH GLYCEMIC INDEX FRUITS (for Protein and Mixed Metabolic Types)

Seriously, ALL of these foods convert to high blood sugar levels in our bodies once they enter our bloodstream. So you must be diligent when eating these types of foods, even if they are being "advertised" as healthy choices for you. The simplest way I know of to get a quick grasp of just how much sugar these products contain is a great conversion trick originated by Dr. Brenda Watson. Through a lifetime of dedication, Brenda has been looking out for us for decades now. Her wealth of experience and knowledge allowed her to bring this magical formula to the forefront of this fight with the Sugar Monsters.

"As the Diva of Digestion, I have always recognized the importance of a healthy diet as a main contributor to digestive health and to total-body health. One of the best ways to improve your diet is to remove sugar. As the 60 Minutes segment illustrates, sugar has the same addictive qualities as cocaine. In fact, they mentioned that people build a tolerance to sugar, always wanting more and more. The result has only been more and more heart disease, diabetes, and cancer. Please, pass this on. Everyone needs to know the harms of sugar." - Brenda Watson

When looking at a food label, simply take the number of grams of carbohydrates listed minus the number of fiber grams and divide that number by five. This will give you a quick and easy idea as to how many teaspoons of sugar are hiding in the food you are about to consume.

Again, it is the number of grams of carbohydrates listed per serving, not the number of grams of sugar listed.

Brenda Watson's Formula:
grams of Carbohydrates - # grams of Fiber ÷ 5 = # of Sugar Teaspoons

It is commonly recommended that you consume no more than 10 teaspoons of total sugar a day. Yet, most people are having twice that with their breakfast alone. **In fact, the average adult consumes over 150 lbs. of sugar a year. Considering there are roughly 96 teaspoons in a pound of sugar, that means the average adult consumes over 14,400 teaspoons of sugar a year by the time the industry sneaks you into their Bermuda Triangle! In the 1700s, people consumed less than eight pounds a year on average. In other words, they had roughly TWO teaspoons of total sugar a day.** And guess what, they survived just fine without it. Yes, the human race can and was intended to survive without boat loads of sugar. This goes for all sugar and its various forms. And please do not start talking that "all-natural" crap to me with regard to sugar. Arsenic is "all natural" and yet one tablespoon will kill you dead. So get over the "it's natural," therefore it must be good for me crap.

And for those food labels that continue to bait you like a big tuna—hook, line, and sinker— claiming that their Bermuda Triangle foods contain "all-natural ingredients," chew on this: secretions from the anal glands of beavers produce a bitter, smelly, orange-brown substance known as castoreum that is used extensively in vanilla and raspberry flavoring. It's legally labeled as "natural flavoring." — The Wild Diet, by Abel James.

Are you beginning to see the problem? Open your eyes and Wake Up!

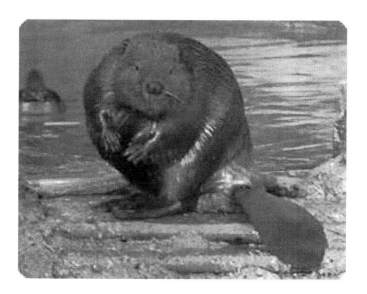

For example, if you are looking at that box of "Bunny Butt Heerios" (not what it is really called—but rhymes with this), this is what you might see:

Nutrition Facts

Serving Size ¾ cup (28g)
Servings Per Container about 17

Amount Per Serving	Honey Nut Cheerios	with ½ cup skim milk
Calories	110	150
Calories from Fat	15	15
	% Daily Value**	
Total Fat 1.5g*	2%	2%
Saturated Fat 0g	0%	0%
Trans Fat 0g		
Polyunsaturated Fat 0.5g		
Monounsaturated Fat 0.5g		
Cholesterol 0mg	0%	1%
Sodium 160mg	7%	9%
Potassium 115mg	3%	9%
Total Carbohydrate 22g	7%	9%
Dietary Fiber 2g	8%	8%
Soluble Fiber less than 1g		
Sugars 9g		
Other Carbohydrate 11g		
Protein 2g		
Vitamin A		

Take a look at this label. As you can clearly see, there are 22 grams of carbohydrates and two grams of fiber per serving. The label also lists nine grams of sugar. However, for our conversion, we are not concerned with grams of sugar. Following our formula, we take the 22 grams of carbs minus our 2 grams of fiber and divide that by 5: 22 - 2 ÷ 5 = 4 teaspoons of sugar. At first glance, one might think this isn't bad; however, most health experts only recommend 10 teaspoons of sugar a day. So, can you imagine having almost half of your daily sugar intake with a measly 110 calories of food? Not to mention, we still haven't added the milk yet. Add milk, and you are now at over half your sugar intake for the whole day. Additionally, the vitamins, minerals, and vital nutrients your body has received are simply subpar. And this is a "healthy alternative" to cereal. Are you starting to get the picture on how and why these processed foods are nothing less than convenient "junk food" with little to no nutritional value? Still think four teaspoons of sugar doesn't sound bad? Ok, try this. Pour yourself a cup of water and take four teaspoons of sugar and add it to the cup. Now stir, and stir...... and stir.....and stir.......still stirring. Now drink it! This is basically what you are getting when you start your day off with a "healthy dose of Bunny Butt Heerios." Come on now, Wake the Fork Up® people! This is anything but a healthy start to our day. The sad fact is that most other cereals are far worse than this.

So, you don't eat cereal? What about that bagel that so many start their day off with? Let's take a look at an average bagel. Look at this label and tell me if you think this is a nutritious start to your day.

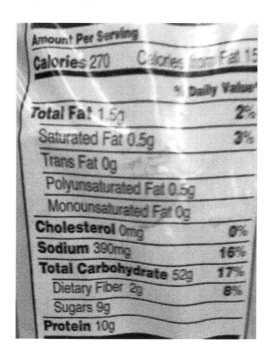

For that good old breakfast bagel you just can't seem to live without, this is what we get. 52 grams of carbohydrates - 2 grams of fiber ÷ 5. **That's 10 teaspoons of sugar to start your day!** Can you imagine some people then add a sugary coffee or juice to this? Do you wonder why the Sugar Monsters begin to take over when you are eating like this? This is only one bagel people. You know what I am going to say next... Wake the Fork Up®. Not only does this cause major imbalances in your body's system, as previously discussed, it also puts fat on you in all the wrong places. Your triglycerides, LDL, and blood pressure suffer directly as a result of this sugar. Your liver, pancreas, and arteries can become damaged as well. This is extremely unhealthy for you, outside of the fact that it sabotages your lean, mean, sexy, fat-burning machine.

Speaking of juices, do you have any idea how the ever so popular orange juice looks under the Intelligent Eating Microscope. Let's take a look:

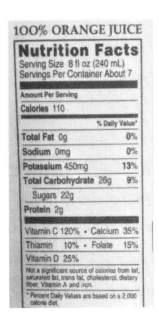

100% ORANGE JUICE

Nutrition Facts

Serving Size 8 fl oz (240 mL)
Servings Per Container About 7

Amount Per Serving

Calories 110

	% Daily Value*
Total Fat 0g	0%
Sodium 0mg	0%
Potassium 450mg	13%
Total Carbohydrate 26g	9%
Sugars 22g	
Protein 2g	

Vitamin C 120%	•	Calcium	35%
Thiamin 10%	•	Folate	15%
Vitamin D 25%			

Not a significant source of calories from fat, saturated fat, trans fat, cholesterol, dietary fiber, Vitamin A and iron.

* Percent Daily Values are based on a 2,000 calorie diet.

Can you say pure sugar? What in the world are people doing loading up with orange juice every morning? Sure the mass media sells it as the vitamin C drink of choice. Believe me, you can get a hell of a lot better food source for vitamin C throughout your day, easily, without annihilating your body with this simple sugar. Some of my favorites are sweet red peppers, green bell peppers, guava, broccoli, brussel sprouts, kiwi, strawberries, and wait for it...a REAL ORANGE. Skip the juices folks, as they are nothing more than glorified sugar.

Are there some carbohydrate sources that don't have fiber that may be ok for us? That is an excellent question and for certain reasons, I say yes. For example, while most yogurt doesn't have fiber and does have some sugar; it is packed with powerful gut-healing nutrients such as probiotics and powerful lean muscle building protein. But, once again, you must step out of the box and think a little more than the average bear when choosing which yogurt to eat. You must continue to develop your Primary Method of Eating.

Let's look at another label, shall we? Let's look at yogurt, for example:

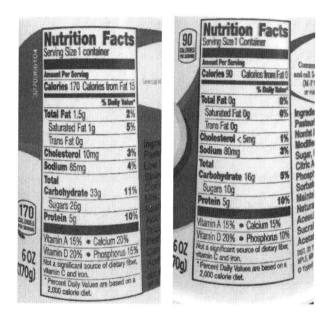

This is how most people eat yogurt...in its highly processed form with loads and loads of sugar. The yogurt on the left shows 33 grams of Carbohydrates - 0 grams of fiber. Put this into our formula: *33 - 0 ÷ 5 and we come up with over 6 and*

a half teaspoons of sugar! Now look at the "light version." We have *16 grams of carbohydrates - 0 grams of fiber ÷ 5 = 3+ teaspoons of sugar in their "healthy light version."* And again, this is with less than 10% of your total daily calories. Do you think you will be able to only consume another seven teaspoons of sugar with the remaining 1,000 plus calories you are to consume over the rest of the day? Highly unlikely. **However, if you simply step into your common sense corner and get the *plain Greek yogurt*, you get a much healthier alternative. Sure there is still some sugar, but it is half to one-third of the other "normal yogurts."**

> *Plus, this yogurt is power packed with muscle-building protein. This protein is extremely important as it drastically decreases the glycemic load, which in turn decreases the blood sugar response tremendously.*

Therefore, your body will be able to utilize these calories for much needed energy as opposed to storing them as fat on your butt, hips, thighs, and belly. Take a look at the next label for plain, fat-free Greek yogurt.

Nutrition Facts

Serving Size 1 Cup (227g)
Servings Per Container 4

Amount/serving	
Calories 130	Fat Cal. 0

	%DV*
Total Fat 0g	0%
Sat. Fat 0g	0%
Trans Fat 0g	
Cholest. 10mg	3%
Sodium 105mg	4%
Total Carb. 11g	4%
Dietary Fiber 0g	0%
Sugars 6g	
Protein 22g	44%

Vitamin A 0% · Vitamin C 0%
Calcium 25% · Iron 0%

*Percent Daily Values (DV) are based on a 2,000 calorie diet.

With just over 2 teaspoons of sugar and 22 grams of protein, Plain Greek Yogurt is not only the best yogurt choice—it is the ONLY choice if you want to maximize fat loss. Understand? Good!

Lastly, we need to have a simple discussion about artificial sweeteners. Most artificial sweeteners are nothing more than chemicals blended together that absolutely have a negative impact on your liver, pancreas, and overall homeostasis of health. Aspartame (NutraSweet, Equal), Sucralose (Splenda) and acesulfame (Sunett) have been linked to other disorders in the body as well. More importantly, these artificial sweeteners can actually raise your blood sugar levels in a similar fashion to normal sugar. In fact, according to research conducted by the Washington University School of Medicine of

St. Louis, sucralose had a high enough impact on blood glucose (blood sugar) to warrant diabetic warnings. Furthermore, according to Dr. Melina Jampolis, who is an internist and physician nutrition specialist, research in both animals and humans suggests the taste of sweet can boost appetite, and also reinforce cravings for and dependence on sugar. In other words, we need to do our best to avoid these artificial sweeteners. If you must have a sweetener in your coffee or tea, it must be natural, and not plain sugar.

My top three favorites are as follows.

1.) Natural Stevia such as SweetLeaf™ (not Truvia or Pure Via, as these are just Coca Cola and Pepsi's chemical-laden versions to trick you once again—they are not pure natural stevia): waketheforkup.com/shop/sweet-leaf/

2.) Natural Xylitol such as Smart Sweet (from organic hardwood, not corn— it is also GMO free, USA): waketheforkup.com/amazon-sweeteners/

3.) Erythritol Natural Blend, such as Lakanto® (Lakanto is a delicious combination of non-genetically modified erythritol and the naturally sweet fruit lo han guo). This is a Great Baking Natural Sweetener Alternative and has no effect on our blood sugar. waketheforkup.com/amazon-sweeteners/

"0 Trans Fats, My Ass"

Now let's talk about another dirty little food industry secret. In 2006, the FDA regulations required *all* foods to list trans fats on the label. However, did you know that they only have to list those foods that have **.5 grams of trans fats per serving** on the labels? So what do you think they do?

Yep, they lower the serving size to a level that gets them under this .5g per serving benchmark and are then able to list their foods as "0 trans fats." In case you have been hiding under a rock, man-made trans fatty acids are bad for us.

I am not talking about the natural trans fats we find in some red meats, which are known as conjugated linoleic acid. This trans fat is fine for us. However, the trans fats they sneak into most processed "on the shelf" foods is atrocious. Very simply, these processed trans fats are vegetable oils given an added hydrogen atom to enable the fat to have a better "solid" shelf life. This is done through a process called hydrogenation.

So *hydrogenated* and partially *hydrogenated oils* are trans fats, and anytime you see this word in the ingredients, you know there is some trans fatty acids in that food, no matter what the label may claim. Where do we find most of these trans fats? Cakes, cookies, chips, French fries, most fried foods in restaurants, and most fast food restaurant items. Remember, they only have to minimize the amount to .5g per serving to say it is trans fat free. The problem is, even at .5g per serving, these fats are very bad for us and will sabotage our fat-burning mechanisms as well. In fact, trans fats have been linked to raising LDL (bad cholesterol) and lowering HDL (good cholesterol), all while triggering inflammation in blood vessels and wreaking havoc on our cardiovascular system. They are also now thought to increase the risk of some cancers.

So what have they used to replace these trans fats in our foods? Besides tropical oils (coconut, palm, and palm kernel) and plant oils (canola, corn, peanut, soy, and sunflower), *they*

148

have created a new Frankenstein food oil called Interesterified fats or IE. Like trans fats, they have chemically altered
fatty acids from liquid oils to solidify them. Early research is
already showing that these have harmful effects on our bodies
as well.

> *So in a word, if you see the words hydrogen-*
> *ated or interesterified on the food label ingredi-*
> *ents section, beware and stay clear. These*
> *foods will NOT get you ripped, lean, and sexy.*

Estrogenic Foods

In a perfect situation, a healthy body will have a nice balance of hormones such as estrogen, leptin, growth hormone,
and testosterone, as previously stated in the book. However,
throwing these hormones out of balance with too much estrogen can wreak havoc on men and women's bodies and result
in disease and disorder followed by massive fat storage. Unbeknownst to many, phytoestrogens and xenoestrogens have
been finding their way into our food sources for some time
now. These estrogenic mimicking compounds in our food and
water pack on unsightly, unhealthy fat in our most troubled
zones such as the belly, low back, hips, buttocks, thighs, and
upper arms (triceps region). Women, you know how you all
hate to have your upper arms wave goodbye before you do.
For men, estrogenic, stubborn fat finds its way to your chest.
Let's face it, moobs (man boobs) are no fun for anyone...just
ask your sex counterpart. Even worse, this fat-forming phenomenon is a self-fulfilling prophecy once it gets started, as
this now "estrogenic fat" increases the rate of accumulation of
even more fat. That's correct; the more estrogen you have
above the normal range, the more fat your body continues to
produce and store. As if this isn't bad enough, this hormone

imbalance has also been linked to many diseases and disorders. As for great sex, this estrogen imbalance will throw your sex life right out the window, as your libido drops down next to nothing. This stuff is bad for you, people. Wake the Fork Up®!

Soy and soy-based products (anything with soy isoflavones) are some of the worst of the food sources. I know that the "food industry" promotes this as "health food," but this is total BS, as the soy in their products has been stripped of all its natural benefits. In fact, by the time soy hits our food source, it is virtually nothing more than estrogenic producing isoflavones such as glycinol, genistein, and daidzein, all of which are nothing short of horrendous for your health, in my professional opinion.

In fact Tulane University recently discovered that glycinol is so "good" at mimicking estrogen that they are concerned with serious complications such as reproductive development and endocrine disruption, as so many other scientists have seen for decades now. So, for starters, stop sucking on the "soy teet" and all the bogus food marketing on how soy is so good for you.

It is utter BS!

Please note that the vast majority of all "health food" *protein products,* such as protein health bars, are filled with this substandard form of protein and are therefore terrible for your fat-burning goals. This is why I only recommend the following for your protein powder and protein bar needs and nutrition. Biotrust™ Low Carb Protein Powder, Biotrust™ protein bars, and Quest Bars are the only three protein supplement sources currently approved by Wake the Fork Up® at this moment. (Of course I recommend the Quest bars that are sucralose free, such as these flavors: cinnamon roll, coconut cashew, lemon cream pie, chocolate peanut butter, and strawberry cheesecake.)

You can order yours here: waketheforkup.com/shop/biotrust-products/biotrust-low-carb/; waketheforkup.com/shop/biotrust-products/biotrust-organic-protein-bars/ and/or waketheforkup.com/shop/quest-nutrition/quest-nutrition-products/.

I like the Quest bars for Protein and Mixed Nutritional types and the Biotrust™ bars for the Carb Nutritional Metabolic Type. Most other protein products will be filled with harmful chemicals and fillers, as well as soy lecithin (soy protein). Stay away from these sources as much as possible, as they will NOT help you burn fat fast.

> *Next, realize that unless your fish, dairy, and meat is wild or organic and grass-fed, more than likely they were given estrogen-producing feed and drugs that will emasculate even a dude like Dwayne "The Rock" Johnson.*

According to The Audubon's Living Oceans Campaign, "farmed salmon are fed more antibiotics per pound of 'livestock' than are any other farmed animal." In fact, 23 million pounds of antibiotics are used annually in US animal production. The Big Food Industry has YOU mislead once again. They actually have folks believing that there are no safe "wild" waters to get our fish from. Why do they do this, you ask? To

Increase Their Bottom Line Profits at the Expense of YOUR Health. Their "farmed fish" is the MOST TOXIC meat on the market today. That's a fact! Get it wild or don't get it at all. And it is no better for most women either, unless you enjoy having flabby arms, asses, and abs. This is why quality of meat is so damn important, people. In other words, eat only wild fish, grass-fed beef, and organic-free range meats if possible. This goes for eggs and cheeses as well. You must eat food that comes from healthy sources, period. Try some of my favorites, provided at TOPLINE and delivered straight to your doorstep, here: waketheforkup.com/shop/topline-foods/.

The same goes for fruits and vegetables that are treated with pesticides and herbicides. These chemicals in our food sources cause fat growth to increase more rapidly than you can imagine. Do your best to shop for locally grown, organic foods. Particularly, to fight against these estrogenic compounds and start burning that tough, stubborn fat today, add avocados, broccoli, brussels sprouts, cabbage, cauliflower, raw nuts (not roasted), and seeds. Also, there are many flavones and flavonones in garlic, onions, raw honey, citrus fruits, chamomile, and passionflower that fight against estrogenic compounds. Make sure they work for your metabolic type, of course. At Wake the Fork Up® we get our healthy nuts from our super food store here: waketheforkup.com/sunfood/.

Lastly, avoid water, soft drinks, and all other plastic bottled liquids and processed foods that are packed in plastic derivatives with harmful chemicals such as BPAs (this is also estrogen mimicking). Again, you find the water "industry" selling you "clean water" packed in fat-producing, chemical-laden, plastic bottles. Many have protested this, so the food industry tried to get one over on you again. You know those bottles they claim to be good for you now, because they are

"BPA FREE"? Most of those BPA free plastic containers you now are drinking from contain equally damaging BPS chemicals that leach into your bloodstream. A 2013 study by Cheryl Watson at The University of Texas Medical Branch at Galveston found that even picomolar concentrations (less than one part per trillion) of BPS can disrupt a cell's normal functioning, which could potentially lead to metabolic disorders such as diabetes and obesity, asthma, birth defects or even cancer. Bad news, peeps. Get yourself a water filter at home and a BPA/BPS-free water bottle that you fill yourself with lean sources of healthy water as often as you can. WE LIKE THIS ONE: waketheforkup.com/shop/amazon-products/life-factory-water-bottle/. Which leads me to the obvious. Do you really think that a 220 pound person needs to only drink the same 64 ounces of water most recommend for everyone? Really? Why in the heck would anyone think a person that weighs 110 pounds would require the same amount of water as someone who weighs 200 plus pounds? This is ridiculous and anyone that steps into their common sense corner could figure this out. Yet, the machine keeps selling you the one-size-fits-all nonsense. Listen, do your best to drink a minimum of .5 ounces of clean water for every pound on your body. If you hit your **DIRT**™ workouts regularly, try to increase this to .75 to 1 ounce per pound. Remember many studies have shown that good ole H_2O increases our metabolism while providing us with our number one nutrient all at the same time. In fact, according to scientists in both Germany and Canada, starting your day out with a chilled glass of water can boost your metabolism up to 30% and lasts nearly 90 minutes after your last sip. You must consume water, folks.

Now listen up, as I do not expect you to change everything at once. It can take days, months, and years to make some of these changes. Do not panic, step into your common sense corner, and take one step forward at a time. In time, these steps add up and you will be well on your way to becoming a WTFU Warrior.

For example, here is a chart that you can use in the beginning to understand which foods you may want to start considering finding better (organic) sources of, as they are the most vulnerable to pesticides and herbicides.

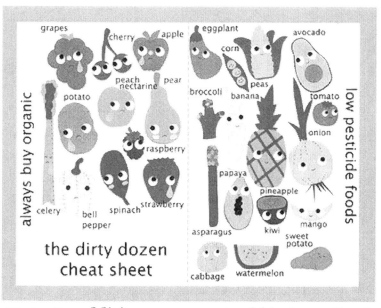

Note: In addition, you must add kale, collard greens, and summer squash to the dirty dozen cheat sheet.

Is it really any wonder why our health care system is in complete and utter disarray? Is it really surprising to you that so many are overweight and undernourished, even in the 21st century? Much of this has been created and perpetuated by the food industry itself. And don't get me started on our government and all their food subsidies for corn, wheat, dairy, etc.! That, in and of itself, is an entire book on its own. But make no mistake people, those of us in the know are consistently and correctly well aware that the government's food guidelines are nothing short of subpar. So please understand, with regard to YOUR body and its specific nutritional needs, many whom you trust are working against you. Not anymore, however. You are becoming a leader and not a follower.

Your "Wake the Fork Up" Call
Many so-called "professionals" are still confused

Many so-called professionals and medical experts would still like you to believe that the formula is quite simple; calories in versus calories out combined with genetics and/or prescriptions. Do you really think walking and talking in a lean, mean, fat-burning body happens simply by performing more exercise and eating less? Do you honestly believe that there is a magic pill that is safe for you that melts away body fat? Do you really believe that all your body's challenges are your parents' fault? Really? Think again Warriors. The reality is that those of us who walk around daily in our best bodies, sporting eight pack abs and sexy glutes, toned thighs, calves, and arms, have known this is a bunch of BS for many, many years now. We know the truth and the secrets to unlocking the fat-burning, high energy vaults, and we practice them. Yet, so many people are still trying to "dumb it down" in order to make you feel like you're simply either eating too much or not exercising enough. Your genetics are "just the way it is" or, even worse, there is a "magic pill" to take.

In fact, I am reminded of a BBQ I attended a few summers back with a friend in Chicago. The host of the BBQ was a very prominent cardiac heart surgeon who, oddly enough, had just finished his first book. As he and I engaged in conversation, his thoughts and focus quickly went to his wife, who was standing in the opposite corner of the deck eating cupcakes at the party. He stated that she had been battling weight problems for many years now and that most of her friends were also heavy. As I glanced over, his statement that most of her friends—who were hovering around the cupcakes, sipping on soft drinks and juices—were very overweight appeared to be accurate. I thought to myself, 'Well, with the poor quality foods they are stuffing their faces with, it's no wonder.' In fact, most of his patients were extremely overweight, he stated. Of course, he knew I was intrigued, and he baited me as well as other guests into this conversation.

As I carefully listened to his discussion, he began to "dumb it down" for the rest of the group, for my girlfriend at the time, and for me (so he thought) as well. She, knowing my passion and intensity for sharing the truth, started to smirk at me as she could feel the "Wake the Fork Up®" moment coming from this measly little kinesiologist (as this prominent heart surgeon was so pompously presenting it), certified strength and conditioning specialist, lifestyle leader and coach, who was in the know and ready to unleash the hounds. As everyone looked upon the good doctor as if he had, yet again, let society off the hook, I took a slow, deep breath and then commanded the attention of his guests with some quick, smart, and easy to follow short solutions and explanations as to what may help her and the others. My explanations were clear and scientifically sound, and yet easy to implement. Some of his guests were beginning to get excited by the topic, as the interest in this corner of the 1100 square foot deck was starting to heat up. While I felt his wife could have clearly benefited from the conversation, although probably not the apropos time for addressing her overweight issues, she was still on the other side of the deck playing host to the other guests at the party.

As I closed my proactive presentation, he had clearly become threatened by my suggestions. This became evident by his next statement. You see, according to him, his wife, her overweight friends, and his overweight patients were simply victims of liking food too much, victims of society, or victims of GOD GIVEN circumstance (genetics). The usual suspects of not having enough time, doesn't like to exercise, has a sweet tooth, eats out too much, cooks too much, has bad genetics, etc. The excuses coming from this cardiologist were endless...he literally covered all the bases for the top 10 excuses on why they were fat and unhealthy. After all, "Look at me, I eat whatever I want, don't exercise, and practically haven't gained a *pound* in over 10 years," he said. Poor poor wife, poor poor patients, and poor poor friends.

What happened next was the first of many uncomfortable exchanges between me and the good doctor. You see, when I began my training in college in 1987 in this field, I was no stranger to fitness, health, and wellness. During summer vacations, friends and I used to work out in the tool shed behind my house every morning. We used the concrete plastic weights for resistance with a run to the water pump and back with intervals. I have recently realized that I had already been "training" myself and others from about the ripe young age of 14. I was also becoming aware that certain foods allowed us to have higher degrees of peak performance with our workouts than others. A keen observation for a 14-year-old. Now, please understand that my 23 years of training experience does not include those years. Also understand that I made tons of mistakes back then and even got completely out of shape and overweight myself, as previously stated. Never the less, some hints to my life's journey were already giving me clues at a very early age, although, at the time, they were unbeknownst to me.

You see, it is my belief that each and every one of us on planet earth have at least *one* thing in this world that we are nearly genius at in life. Some are near genius level at more than one thing, but most are geniuses of at least *one* thing. What the good doctor didn't realize is that my genius, my 10,000 plus hours of concentration, was on being a biomechanical, health and fitness guru, specialist of sorts. As a result, not only do I love what I do, but I look at my work and people with a slightly different approach than most. No, I don't see dead people, but I do possess some sort of a sixth sense when it comes to sizing a person up. You see, part of my "near genius, 10,000 hour focus" includes an ability to take a look at most any person and be able to tell them their body fat percentage within plus or minus three percent. I am not always right with this, but nearly always. So, while the good doctor appeared, to most, to be healthy and lean, to me, I could easily tell that his body fat was roughly 25 percent or higher, as he was what we call "fat but skinny." Now, for a woman in her 40's and up, this would not be considered elite, or a WTFU Warrior, but it would not necessarily be viewed as unhealthy. However, for a man, this is downright unhealthy, not to mention unattractive, had he taken his shirt off. So, not only did I inform him that just because he hadn't "gained a pound" in nearly 10 years and could eat almost anything, that he wasn't necessarily healthy. Not to mention, his strength, flexibility, functional physical performance, and overall fitness level was clearly subpar.

> *But, oh yes, I did...I informed him that at nearly 25 percent body fat, he was not only unfit, but clearly was placing unnecessary risk on many of his body's critical systems, including...his heart! This cardiologist asked for it, and he got it, people.*

The conversation slowed quickly, and the subject was changed, but I later heard, through the grapevine, that he had his body fat measured and it was...wait for it...27 percent. Supposedly, he is looking into "better ways" to improve his health and fitness. I have not had contact with him since, however, so I am unsure as to the validity of my "inside information." I wish him well, and encourage him to stop dumbing things down and stretch his knowledge muscles when it comes to guiding his patients and himself.

I have had the pleasure of working with many doctors, surgeons, PhDs, and other health professionals over the years. And many of them are clearly intelligent, capable people who are performing admirable services. In fact, one of my past clients and now good friend, Dr. Bernie Wetchler, was literally one of the leading pioneers in his medical specialty, a man of true integrity and a wealth of knowledge. My personal physician, Lou, is also a fine medical team member who looks at all the possible avenues to bettering his patients' health and wellness. And many of my friends are practicing medicine in some of the most advanced, proactive manners to date.

However, plenty of health care professionals do not practice healthy lifestyles and even more have absolutely no concept of solid nutrition, exercise physiology, and lifestyle management. And why would they? Their medical training covers less than 40 hours of focus in this area, with an average of 19.6 contact hours in the focus of nutrition. Not to mention, many doctors and health care specialists are in bed with the big pharmaceutical companies. They find ways to get compensated for "selling" pharmaceutical companies' drugs. In fact, every major drug company has armies of "pharmaceutical reps" out there, every single day, peddling their products to these doctors...beautiful young women, and some men, who could sell a turkey baster to a vegetarian, if they needed to. I know, as I have dated a few women who did this and these ladies were hot and damn good at selling things. So, don't always think that the medical field has your best interests at heart. I'm not saying that all doctors are bad. I am simply stating that medical care is a business, people. This is simply a fact, so Wake Up.

Your "Wake the Fork Up" Call
All Calories are not created equal

Along the same lines as previously stated, many people continue to walk down the wrong path regarding this topic as well. It is amazing to me how people wouldn't dare place diesel fuel into their non-diesel cars and expect the car to run properly. After all, 20 gallons of gas is 20 gallons of gas, right? Wrong, as your car would barely last a week on that fuel, let alone make it a block for some vehicles. So why do you think that you can feed yourself any kind of food and have your body perform properly, so long as it is within the right "calorie amount"? Does this make any sense to you?

Now, I am assuming by now that most of you realize that one gram of carbohydrate, and one gram of protein is equivalent to four calories. And that one gram of fat is measured as nine calories. Did you know that the body processes one gram of alcohol as seven calories? Did you know that your body has a completely different response internally depending on the type of foods that you eat? For example, 300 calories of white bread would most likely be stored as fat on your body versus the same 300 calories being a nice cut of salmon? Even though the salmon clearly has a higher percentage of fat. Did you know that your body has certain foods that it prefers that could be completely different from those preferred by your neighbors, brother, partner, or kids?

It's true, as science shows us that you have a nutritional metabolic type that allows your body to process 300 calories of some foods much better than it processes 300 calories of other foods. Did you know that you have a very distinct metabolic type that determines how one man's food can be another man's poison? Did you know that every single item we put into our mouths has some sort of blood sugar response and that, based on that response, your body will either store the food as fat, or utilize it efficiently and effectively for energy and other vital requirements? The glycemic load is very real and very important in that same 300 calories. Did you know that our foods (fuel) consist of many micronutrients made up of vitamins, minerals, and trace elements that allow our bodies to burn more or less fat? Not to mention, combining these foods with other foods allows us to better absorb and utilize these micronutrients better than others. Have your blueberries with a dairy product and receive less of the valuable nutrients than you would having those same 100 calories of blueberries in combination with another lean protein. It's true. Other foods raise our body's natural thermogenesis (body heat), enabling us to burn more calories as fat and energy versus storing them.

The list goes on and on people, and I want you to know that once you figure this formula out, you will literally be able to consume more of the right calories and burn more and more fat. In fact, oftentimes, those individuals who take in too few calories on the "starvation diets" end up altering their metabolism and storing even more body fat. Food science and nutrition performance has come a long, long way people. To walk around and allow yourself to be "dumbed down" by thinking all calories are equally healthful is archaic and ridiculous. This is your "wake up" moment, and I am here to tell you that this book will clear all of this up for you, once and for all. You will be armed and dangerous when it comes to your attack on fat. You will become a leader in this arena and not a follower.

*The truth about food is that it is absolutely the fuel that drives our bodies to either living lives of blissful, healthful harmony filled with lean, ripped bodies performing at optimal levels, or living less than average **dis**eased and **dis**ordered lives complicated with many undesirable responses and reactions.*

There is an optimal way to fuel your body and in order to do so, you must first truly understand the basics. I realize that this book is primarily designed to help your body burn fat while keeping lean, toned muscle. However, the more you understand this system, the leaner you will be, I assure you. So, stick with me as I not only teach you the best way to get ripped, but also the healthiest way to keep all your vital systems performing optimally for you.

MACRONUTRIENTS: YOUR NUTRITIONAL BUILDING BLOCKS

By now, most of you have heard of the three macronutrients known as protein, carbohydrates, and fats. They are the essential building blocks of all the foods we consume and, therefore, get a fair amount of attention in our media today. Most foods consist of all three macronutrients, but we generally refer to foods as belonging to only one of these groups. For example, most people think of eggs, meat, fish, and dairy as sources of protein. Nuts, oils, and cheeses are often thought of as fats, whereas breads, grains, fruits, and vegetables are generally thought of as carbohydrates. This is because, while many of these foods have all three macronutrients, they *predominantly* have one of the three.

Taking our example, a walnut has a general nutritional breakdown as follows: 90% fat, 6% protein, and 4% carbohydrates. So, we naturally refer to this source of food as a fat. A nice cut of lean, boneless, skinless chicken breast is roughly 90% protein, 10% fat, and 0% carbohydrates. We naturally refer to this as a protein. And the average slice of bread is roughly 75% carbohydrates, 20% protein, and 5% fat, although we all reference bread as being a carbohydrate. Yet, most foods consist of a combination of the groups. Oftentimes, foods will have much closer percentages and are often referred to as one group, when in fact they have more concentration of another group. This happens a lot with packaged and processed foods, and it can become confusing. It can also happen with some healthier foods as well, such as many yogurts. They are generally considered to be a protein source, but oftentimes, depending on the yogurt, have more fat and/or carbohydrates than protein. So, it is important that you understand, that for the purpose of this book, I will be referring to such foods in relation or relevance to what they are comprised of most.

It is equally important that you understand the power of protein. Proteins, very simply, are essential for anabolic muscle building, hormone production, carrying nutrients throughout the body, and cellular regeneration and repair, to name just a few. The skinny on fat is simply this: it is requisite for healthy brains, sex hormone regulation, healthy hair and skin, and providing cushion for our organs, plus much more. As for the carbohydrate controversy, one needs their daily carb intake for such vital things as energy production, proper cellular metabolism in our brain, and red blood cells, just to name a few. However, the key is to get the right carbs, fats, and proteins and the right amounts of them for your unique metabolic type.

CHAPTER ELEVEN
Determining Your Nutritional Metabolic Type

"The food that you eat can either be the safest & most powerful form of medicine, or the slowest form of poison."

—*Ann Wigmore*

Step One: YOUR Nutritional Metabolic Type

I have already alluded to the fact that you have a unique nutritional metabolic type.

This type is so important, and it's absolutely the reason why some people are able to get great results in fat loss, sexual function, and a general sense of well-being eating one style of nutrition while others get lousy results eating the same foods.

And when it comes to burning fat, what other nutrition program could you think of being more important than a program designed specifically for YOUR **nutritional metabolic type**? I can't think of a single one, and in fact, in over 23 years of practice, I can honestly say that this nutrition program produces phenomenal results. How can I say this?

Easily, as Nutritional Metabolic Typing is the culmination of over 80 years of pioneering efforts and discoveries by a

whole series of remarkable medical researchers including bi-
ochemists, clinical nutritionists, dentists, psychologists, phy-
sicians, and physiologists, many of whom are world renowned
in their area of specialty. Dr. George Watson, William Donald
Kelley, Dr. Royal Lee, Dr. Weston Price, Dr. Francis Potten-
ger, Dr. Melvin Page, Dr. Roger Williams, Dr. Emanuel Reici,
Dr. Henry Bieler, William Wolcott, and Trish Fahey—each
and every one of these exceptional individuals poured their
heart, mind, and souls into this research, and we are very for-
tunate to be the benefactors of such a wealth of knowledge.

There are actually nine fundamental homeostatic controls
that determine our metabolic type. Your oxidative system, au-
tonomic nervous system, catabolic/anabolic balance, endocrine type, acid/alkaline balance, prostaglandin balance, con-
stitutional type, electrolyte balance, and blood type. However,
the oxidative system plays the most critical role in managing
the body's metabolic activities and fat-burning abilities, and
in turn, in maintaining health. It is this system more than any
other that determines a person's dietary requirements.
Therefore, it is this system that this book focuses on.

In general, your oxidative system determines the relative
speed at which your cells metabolize carbohydrates. Energy
conversion at the cellular level is a multistep process that requires specific nutrients at each step of the way, says Wolcott
and Fahey (2000). So, your metabolic type absolutely determines the amount and types of proteins, fats, and carbohydrates that you must have in order to have optimal health and
wellness. More importantly, for our goals, eating right for
your nutritional metabolic type is the sneaky little key that un-
locks your fat-burning furnace. Without this key, your results
will never surface.

With this key, your Ryan Gosling and Mila Kunis body is just around the corner. Are you willing to learn what it takes to get your key?

This is why the "one-size-fits-all" diet frenzy is another myth I am debunking, once and for all. You cannot expect every person to eat the exact same way and get the exact same results. Any person with any common sense should know this, as we all have had that friend or family member that can "eat whatever they want" and not gain an ounce. But in actuality, they are not eating whatever they want; they are simply eating those things that you cannot (and therefore want), yet it is right for their body type. Come on now, Wake up People. This nutrition program will set you straight, once and for all.

The first thing we must do is determine what Nutritional Metabolic Type YOU are. The test is very simple and takes less than 10 minutes to complete.

The key, however, is to answer the questions as you really feel, not as you think I (or anyone else, for that matter) would want you to answer. Take a moment to think about each question, and then answer it as best as you can. You will notice that you only have two choices. You must choose one or the other. There will be some questions that have more than one answer that applies to you. Again, you must choose only ONE answer. Choose the one that makes the MOST sense. The one that you absolutely would prefer over the other. It is ok if you normally would not choose either. However, you must choose one. So, if you had to choose one, which one would it be? For some of you, this will be quite simple. For many, however, you rarely think at all about what you eat and why. So, do your best with the test, and then come back and take it a week later just to reevaluate. There is no harm in taking a week to truly listen to your body and its hints as you go throughout your day deciding on what to eat and how you feel before and after consuming the food.

YOUR Metabolic typing test: Modified from *The Metabolic Typing Diet* (Wolcott and Fahey 2000, 135-158). Please note that you will only choose the answer that you would most likely choose, having ONLY the two choices listed.

Taste of Life; An Intellectual Eating Plan™ Nutritional Metabolic Type Test:

1.) For breakfast, I ideally enjoy and feel best if I eat,
a. fruit, cereal, and milk, and/or toast
b. eggs, bacon, ham, and/or sausage

2.) I am most happy and feel my best,
a. when the weather is hot
b. when the weather is colder outside

3.) Most people like sweets to some degree, but ideally if I could only have one or the other, I would choose
a. a nice sweet dessert after a meal
b. a nice snack like popcorn, chips, or cheese

4.) In general, I feel best if I eat,
a. one to three meals per day
b. at least three meals a day with several snacks

5.) If I have sweets right before bed, I generally feel,
a. the sweets do not affect my sleep at all
b. the sweets do not allow for my best sleep right before bedtime

6.) *When experiencing a busy day, skipping meals makes me feel,*
a. *just fine, as I often skip meals*
b. *ñot good at all (tired, no energy, irritable)*

7.) *Contrary to many popular diet programs, fats may not be as bad for us as many would like us to believe. If I could take away the judgment placed upon it, I think that,*
a. *I really don't desire fatty foods.*
b. *1 would eat more of them if they were good for me, as I enjoy them*

8.) *It seems when I gain weight, I usually seem to overindulge on*
dulge on
a. *meats and fatty foods*
b. *breads, pasta, fruits, and juices*

9.) *When I want a lasting energy boost, I usually have success by going for*
a. *candy, pastries, or fruit*
b. *meat and cheese*

10.) *If I am having a day where I feel irritated and anxious, I prefer*
a. *fruits or vegetables or sugary foods to help ease the anxiety*
ety
b. *heavier foods with some fat like nuts with salt and/or meats*

11.) *If I am out celebrating something very special and can eat whatever I want, no holds barred, I prefer to have*
a. *chicken and turkey, salads, fruits and vegetables, and various sweet desserts*

b. ribs, pork chops, potatoes and gravy, salmon and a salad loaded with cheese, and a rich creamy dessert

12.) When I consume coffee, tea, or other drinks with caffeine, I feel
a. pretty good in general
b. a little nervous, hyper, jittery, or hungry

13.) During my usual day, I feel hungry
a. not that often, and in general do not have a big appetite
b. more than most and prefer to eat many times per day

14.) But if I do get hungry during my day, I generally feel best if I eat
a. something sweet
b. cheese and nuts

15.) When I wake up in the morning, I am
a. not that hungry to be honest
b. willing and able to eat

16.) By the time lunch rolls around, I
a. sometimes need to be reminded to eat
b. am hungry and ready to eat my lunch

17.) If I decide to eat sugary snacks, I feel
a. just fine and have newfound energy that lasts
b. a rush of energy, but often crash a little later and don't feel so great after

18.) When I finish a workout or high energy activities, I feel
a. better if I have a high sugary drink such as Gatorade or fruit juice

b. better if I have a protein shake or food high in protein

19.) If I show up at my office and there are salty snacks versus sugary snacks, I
a. am not very interested and wish the snack was a sugary treat
b. jump right in and enjoy the snack

20.) In general, when I think of red meat, I could
a. leave it
b. take it

21.) When I am craving a snack and have both options, I generally choose
a. breads, crackers, cookies
b. peanuts, popcorn, chips

22.) When I think of sour foods, I generally feel that I
a. don't like them
b. like them

23.) I tend to be more
a. of a loner or introvert
b. of a social butterfly

24.) If I had a fruit bowl for lunch, more than likely I would feel
a. more than satisfied until dinnertime
b. irritable, tired, and as if I wanted to eat more shortly afterward

25.) When I feel my best, I am generally

a. *eating only one to three meals daily with little to no snacks*

b. *eating smaller meals & snacks more frequently through-out the day*

Now simply tally up how many A's, and how many B's you have.

My A totals _8_____ My B totals _17_____

According to your totals, if your A score is 5 or more points higher than your B score, then you are a Carb Type. If your B score is 5 or more points higher than your A score, then you are a Protein Type. However, if your A and B scores are within 3 points of one another (example: A=13 and B=12), then you are a Mixed Type.

So, to make it easy, if you Score 15 or above on A, you are a Carb Type.

If you score 15 or above on B, you are a Protein Type.

If your score is less than 15 on both A and B, you are a Mixed Type.

Congratulations! If you took the time to answer each question honestly, you now know your Nutritional Metabolic Type.

For many, it may have been difficult for you to truly answer the questions, as you rarely take the time to think about what kinds of foods make you feel a certain way. It is ok to take the next three to seven days to start listening to your body, and how you feel after these meals and snacks, and then retake the test.

Now that you have finished, are you surprised at just how easy it was? You are one step closer to being a Greek God/Goddess-like specimen.

> *In fact, once you learn how to eat according to your nutritional metabolic type, not only will your clothes begin to fit better and those swimsuits look amazing on you, but you will start to feel more energized and alive. This is exactly how your body wants to feel naturally.*

This program is specifically for YOU. Are you beginning to get excited? You should be. Included in my ***Taste of Life; An Intellectual Eating Plan***™ are all the details on exactly how, what, and when you should eat according to YOUR Nutritional Metabolic Type. Believe me when I say it does NOT involve counting calories. It does NOT have you adding up points and it will most definitely not have you eating five to six small meals a day. It will, however, have you losing from three to seven pounds of fat within the first week. It will crush your cravings in 72 hours or less. It will be as easy as one, two, three. Go here to get your ***Taste of Life; An Intellectual Eating Plan***™ and start burning fat today: waketheforkup.com/programs/.

CHAPTER TWELVE

Taste of Life: An Intellectual Eating Plan

A Nutrition Plan Tailored Specifically for YOU!

"What I've enjoyed most, though, is meeting people who have a real interest in food and sharing ideas with them. Good food is a global thing and I find that there is always something new and amazing to learn—I love it!"

—Jamie Oliver

Step Two: An Intellectual Eating Plan

It turns out that WHEN we eat is equally as important as what we eat. Much research has consistently been written on this, and many books have popped up in the last few years about this phenomenon. Most of these writings have focused on dietary fasting (no eating for a certain period of time) as a way to minimize calories, fat storage, and hormonal imbalances. Remember, everyone fasts to some extent every time we go to sleep, hence the word breakfast (first meal of the day "breaks" the "fast"). Some suggest that you not eat for periods of 20 to 48 hours at a time. This style of dieting has become known as IF or Intermittent Fasting. However, for many people, the impracticality of not eating for days at a time seriously limits the success rate of such programs. No one doubts that fasting increases your natural production of growth hormone and limits your calories on average, but who wants to go two days without eating?

However, much research has now shown that structured fasting also increases your leptin and insulin sensitivity (this is great for our overall health and fat-burning furnace). The more insulin and leptin sensitive we are, the more our bodies take to fat burning. Structured Intellectual Eating does increase growth hormone, while reducing ghrelin (your "I'm hungry" hormone). Remember, the more growth hormone we have, the more lean muscle and less fat on our bodies. Structured Intellectual Eating does decrease inflammation, and many of the diseases and disorders associated with internal inflammation. This is all really great news, as we are now discovering that YOUR Intellectual Eating Window has a profound impact on your fat-burning furnace and overall health.

As more and more interest accumulates, so does the significance and funding for more research. Consequently, in 2012, Satchidananda Panda and his associates from the internationally renowned Salk Institute for Biological Studies in La Jolla, California confirmed that limiting your "eating/feeding window" on a regular basis had massive benefits on health and wellness, especially with regard to fat metabolism. **That is to say, when their test participants were given a window of opportunity to eat for a specified period of hours per 24-hour cycle (one full day), they lost on average 28% more fat than their counterparts who were allowed to eat the exact same food in the exact same caloric amount, anytime throughout the day. Even more surprising was that the quality of the food was over 60% fat.**

"This was a surprising result," says Megumi Hatori, a postdoctoral researcher in Panda's laboratory and a first author of the study. "For the last 50 years, we have been told to reduce our calories from fat and to eat smaller meals and snacks throughout the day. We found, however, that fasting time is important. By eating in a time-restricted fashion, you can still resist the damaging effects of a high-fat diet, and we did not find any adverse effects of time-restricted eating when eating healthy food." In other words, if for some reason you have to eat those foods that aren't so great for you, utilizing a specified eating window to feed would significantly help with losing unwanted fatty weight. Really exciting news, indeed.

In fact, the study declared that when we fast, the body starts to burn fat and break down cholesterol. On the contrary, when eating frequently all day (like the "one-size-fits-all" five to six small meals a day plans), the body continues to store fuel as fat, "ballooning" fat particularly in the liver cells, which becomes very damaging over time. Also, with Timed Intellectual Eating (timed fasting and eating intervals), the body naturally produces bile via the breakdown of cholesterol that activates Brown Adipose Tissue or BAT. This super fat is the good fat our bodies need and desire, as it is very metabolically active and burns the White Adipose Tissue or nasty, ugly fat hanging around on our bodies. It was also discovered that glucose production from the liver was temporarily shut down, benefitting our DNA through cellular repair and decreasing overall inflammation in the body. Of course, this study only reinforced what many other studies, and clients I have worked with, experienced.

Take, for example, another study cited in the *American Journal of Clinical Nutrition* in 2007. It took a group of participants and fed them the exact same amount of food as well, allowing one group to eat their food three times over the entire course of the day whenever they liked. The other group only had one meal in a restricted time frame. Of course, the group in the restricted time frame (an intellectual eating window) lost significantly more fat, even though they ate the exact same food with the exact same calorie count. In other words, this study only further reinforced what many of us in the know had already suspected; limiting the time window that you allow yourself to eat each and every day has a massive effect on burning excess fat. Similar studies continue to show that shrinking your daily eating window (going without eating for longer periods) also reduces one's risk of diabetes, cardiac disease, and many forms of cancer. In fact, the University of Utah discovered that those individuals who fasted just one day per month decreased their risk of clogged arteries by 40%. This was just one day of intellectual eating a month! These are huge reasons why we must learn the simple yet specific art of *Intellectual Eating*™.

I can hear many of you right now. "But Gary, I thought all the top professionals in the field from here to China have been telling us to eat five to six smaller meals per day or about every two to three hours? Also, isn't breakfast the MOST important meal of the day?" Well, I must confess, I was totally wrong with this assumption, as were so many others in giving you this advice. In fact, studies are now showing us that this continued feeding all day long is throwing off our fat metabolism, while not allowing mitochondria in our liver to burn fat. Again, for a short period of time, even I had it totally wrong. Breakfast is nothing more than "breaking a fast." We just need to have it a good bit later than most of us have been having it for years now. How long are we talking about? This absolutely depends on your nutritional metabolic type. I have calculated all the work for you, right down to the exact minute and the results for my participants have been nothing short of amazing. **Not only do you learn the exact foods to eat for your body type, but I show you exactly when to eat these delicious foods and over how many meals.**

I tell you exactly when you can start eating for the day and exactly when you need to call it a day. Guess what? It is NOT the same for everyone. It also does not involve you trying to fast for 24-48 hours. That is just impractical and therefore never works. You will eat more normally than most. I guarantee it. You must learn this in order to get your best results.

One huge bonus—exercising before your intellectual eating window begins has actually been shown to increase our natural growth hormone, insulin sensitivity, and leptin sensitivity.

In fact, one study actually produced an increase of 1300% for women and 2000% for men with growth hormone, according to the Intermountain Medical Center Heart Institute! This is your "fountain of youth" hormone, and it will literally turn your body into a fat-burning machine.

Not to mention imbuing you with beautiful hair, nails, skin, muscle tone, and many other benefits. So, not only has Intellectual Eating been proven to get you the fastest fat-burning results ever, but it also drastically increases the efficiency of your hormonal balance and overall health. What are you waiting for? Get this program today: waketheforkup.com/programs/.

Step Three: Spend less time in "The Bermuda Triangle of Foods"

Remember earlier in your Wake the Fork Up® segment where we discussed The Bermuda Triangle of Foods? These are the foods that literally will make good health and wellness disappear—processed foods filled with sugars, trans fatty acids, and estrogenic producing compounds and chemicals. Unfortunately, this is 80% of most foods in the grocery store. **Don't panic, peeps, as there are currently over 600,000 food choices available. Twenty percent still leaves you with over 100,000 choices. The average person consumes the same 100 foods a year, on average.** So, suggesting you don't have enough foods to choose from is just BS (a belief system that no longer serves you...bullshit). Just try to conduct 80% of your shopping in the outer aisles of the grocery store (this is where fresh meats, Greek yogurt, fresh fruits, and vegetables are sold in the store). This will keep you in a safe zone. Also, remember, if the food industry is offering you half-truths and flat-out lies on how healthy their products are, simply utilize our easy to follow guidelines.

Brenda Watson's Formula: How much Sugar is REALLY in it?
 # grams of Carbohydrates - # grams of Fiber ÷ 5 = # of Sugar Teaspoons

TRY YOUR BEST TO GET NO MORE THAN 10-20 TEASPOONS OF SUGAR A DAY depending on YOUR Nutritional Metabolic Type

Hydrogenated and **Partially Hydrogenated oils** are trans fats.
They have created a new Frankenstein food oil called
Interesterified fats or IE.
Avoid foods that contain these words in the label, EVEN if they say trans fat free

Estrogen Mimicking Foods are to be avoided *as much as possible.*
No soy, plastic container foods/drinks or pesticides
Eat more broccoli, cauliflower, avocados, raw nuts, & organic foods

One particular bonus worth noting. The National Weight Control Registry—an ongoing research project tracking more than 3,000 people who've lost an average of 66 pounds and kept it off for five years—found that keeping a food journal is the one strategy used by the majority of successful dieters. In fact, in a study of 1,685 dieters conducted by a health insurance company, *the best predictor of weight loss throughout the first year was the number of food records kept per week.* Another recent study published in the *American Journal of Preventive Medicine* found that dieters who tracked their food intake in a "food diary" lost twice as much weight as those who didn't track their food. This is according to Rebecca Pratt, a contributing writer to *Spark People.* My favorite food journal is a free app called "MyFitnessPal." It will literally allow you to enter your ***Taste of Life: An Intellectual Eating Plan*™** foods, amounts, etc. and help keep YOU on track. Once in MyFitnessPal.com, Go to Settings > Goals > Change Goals > Custom and put your Macro Nutrient Figures as indicated for your Nutritional Metabolic Type, according to the ***Taste of Life; An Intellectual Eating Plan*™.** Remember, in order to get YOUR customized Nutrition Plan, you must get it here: waketheforkup.com/programs/.

BONUS—The Biotrust™ Difference
Fat Burning Supplements that Actually Work

As a leader in this industry whose life's work has involved finding the very best ways to increase one's ability to walk, talk, and be the very best person they can be, I am always asked one simple question: "Do supplements really work?" To which I carefully respond, "Absolutely, just so you are getting exactly what you pay for and using the few that actually do what they claim to do." In other words, when taken in addition to a sound eating and exercise lifestyle, supplements can in fact enhance your results significantly.

What do you think the problem may be? Yes, once the big corporations discover that significant research has proven that these precious nutrients are good for us, they want to find a way to exploit that information to increase their profits. They then do anything and everything to reduce the quality nutrients needed through substandard processing, below average compounds, and unnecessary fillers. Fillers, you ask? Yes, fillers, such as wood bark and saw dust, as they can legally put up to a certain percentage of these in your supplements. With substandard processing, much like the big food industry, they can actually give you rancid, spoiled nutrients as well. The list really goes on and on, as it is much cheaper for them to pay the fines should they get caught (they rarely get caught, however) than it is for them to do it the right way, which would entail proper processing, nutrients, and labeling. So you must understand that there are very few supplements on the planet that meet or exceed my stringent guidelines. I have been taking and recommending high quality supplements for the past 14 years and the list is very short.

Protein Powders, Bars and BCAAs

For example, we have long known that quality blends of **Protein Powders** and **Branch Chain Amino Acids (BCAAs)** dramatically increase protein synthesis. This, in return, allows the body to keep, build, and tone lean muscle much more effectively than those who do not supplement. But did you know that most of the "health food protein sources" are filled with substandard estrogen-producing soy protein isolates? Did you know that they are also filled with chemicals as well? They are essentially no better for you than a "glorified candy bar." While positioned as "healthy," these fat loss and health-derailing nightmares are full of **simple sugars, damaged and denatured fats, dirt-cheap and unhealthy protein**, and a slew of **artificial colors, sweeteners, and preservatives**. Believe me, these are not supplements *Wake the Fork Up*® Warriors are taking and neither should you. You need a protein source that is filled with only the very best ingredients each and every time. The only protein source supplements that are *Wake the Fork Up*® approved are as follows. **Biotrust™ Low Carb Protein, Biotrust™ Protein Bars and Quest Bars**.

You can find yours here: waketheforkup.com/shop/biotrust-products/biotrust-low-carb/; waketheforkup.com/shop/biotrust-products/biotrust-organic-protein-bars/; waketheforkup.com/shop/quest-nutrition/.

As for the BCAAs, most found on the shelves contain toxic fillers. Remember, BCAAs are essential amino acids your body must get from other sources, as your body will not produce them on its own. This becomes very important as we are leaning out to ensure we only burn fat, and not valuable muscle. Therefore, we only recommend this BCAA source:

waketheforkup.com/shop/biotrust-products/bcaa-matrix/.
It gives you exactly what your body needs every time.

Healthy Omega Fatty Acids—Not the Usual Suspects—OmegaKrill 5X

Significant research has proven that taking **Omega fatty acid blends** (commonly referred to as fish oil) can have a profound effect on the body for brain function, decreasing inflammation, and improving your cardiovascular health. This is because it counterbalances the typical 25:1 ratio of Omega 6 fatty acids to Omega 3 fatty acids we find in the common eating style of today. We actually need the balance to be closer to a 1:1 ratio, so we must supplement with more Omega 3 fatty acids.

What do you think happened when big food and supplement companies got involved? Well, most people on the planet suddenly rushed to the local store to buy substandard forms of this supplement. Seriously, you can find fish oil in any grocery or supplement store today, and the price can be astonishing low for some brands. Why do you think this is? Do YOU really think that these companies have a better process and product that allows them to sell you their brand for so much cheaper? Really?

It is estimated that nearly 90% of the Omega-3 fatty acids contained in traditional fish oil supplements will go unabsorbed by your body's cells, having no positive impact on your health. The two most important types of Omega-3 fatty acids, providing the vast majority of health benefits, are **EPA and DHA.** A comprehensive study performed by Dr. Opperman of the Department of Agriculture and Food Science found that more than half of the fish oil products on the market did not contain the amount of EPA and DHA stated on the label. This same study by Dr. Opperman also discovered that the majority of fish oil products on the market had **higher rancidity levels than vegetable oil (one of the most rancid oils on the shelf).** You see, rancid oil is **extremely inflammatory** and will actually cause much more **damage to your heart,** skin, joints and overall health by taking it. In essence, by buying these products you are PAYING to put your health in danger. You still think that the fish oil you are buying at Wally World is benefiting you? Get a clue. You have been bamboozled once again by the machine. Time to wake up and become a leader, not a follower. Our Omega Krill 5X is the BEST on the planet, guaranteed. The list as to why is very long and very clear cut. Want to learn more? Go here: waketheforkup.com/shop/biotrust-products/omegakrill-5x/.

Healthy Belly FAT Burner—The Best CLA on the Planet

One of the biggest supplements to help aid in burning belly fat is **CLA.** Just how effective is conjugated linoleic acid at burning fat and slimming your waist? In a double-blind, placebo-controlled human study (the gold standard of research design) published in the *Journal of International Medical Research,* 20 participants were either given conjugated linoleic acid or an impostor (in the form of vegetable oil) daily for 12 weeks. At the end of the study period, the **conjugated linoleic acid group lost 20% of their body fat** while the placebo group lost no fat at all. In another double-blind, placebo-controlled human study conducted by renowned Swedish researcher Dr. Annika Snedman, **those receiving conjugated linoleic acid lost 400% more fat than the placebo group** over the course of 12 weeks—and this was all done without any change in diet and without the implementation of a regular exercise program. A third study conducted at the University of Barcelona, Spain measuring the effects of conjugated linoleic acid intake in 60 healthy men and women age 35 to 65 found that subjects receiving conjugated linoleic acid lost significant body fat **(78% of which was from the belly region)** while the placebo group actually GAINED weight. But of course you must get what you actually pay for. The only way I know how to guarantee this is to have you get yours here: waketheforkup.com/shop/biotrust-products/bellytrim-xp/. The usual suspects you find in the "super supplement stores" will not even come close to this quality. It's a fact, Warriors... don't let them confuse you.

LeptiBurn™—*the Key to Continuing Fat Loss*

Remember how important the hormone **Leptin** is for Fat Burning? Some believe this to be one of the most important, if not the most important, hormones for burning fat. The trouble is, the more we restrict our calories and burn the fat, the less leptin our bodies have. This can dramatically slow our fat-burning furnace down by as much as 50% in as little as seven days according to much research. Now, I hate to continue to be the bearer of bad news, but the scenario I just explained is only **half** the problem. The other unfortunate reality is that the vast majority of people are suffering from "leptin resistance" due to years of high body fat levels and a diet full of processed foods. So, of course, my ***Taste of Life; An Intellectual Eating Plan***™ encourages super leptin loading days. However, you want to know the very best and easiest way to guarantee you have enough leptin to keep burning the fat?

What if I told you there was a simple way to support healthy leptin levels as you lose weight, *while also* supporting increased sensitivity to the hormone? Is that something you might be interested in? You see, if you *could* do that, you could essentially keep your body in a fat-burning state **all the**

time... high leptin levels equal high levels of fat burning... 24 hours a day, seven days a week. Can you just imagine how much more fat you'd burn if your body was no longer limiting your rate of fat loss on a daily basis?

Well, it can be done by taking this super supplement— LeptiBurn™: waketheforkup.com/shop/biotrust-products/leptiburn/.

Keeping Your Blood Sugar Controlled—IC 5

Remember what happens when our **Insulin levels** are out of balance? This is why processed carbohydrates are so damaging for so many of us. However, there is a synergistic blend of five compounds that can significantly help you control your insulin levels. Cinnamomum Burmannii, Berberine, Pterocarpus Marsupium, 4-hydroxyisoleucine, and R-Alpha-Lipoic-Acid or simply R-ALA. This supplement is so powerful that it actually helps you to burn fat, instead of store it, even when you consume some not so friendly cautious carbohydrates. This happens for a few reasons—minimum insulin release, quick and efficient blood sugar clearance, and maximum glycogen uptake. In other words, people who take this supplement find they are not as sensitive to the "bad carbs." Test drive this supplement here: waketheforkup.com/shop/biotrust-products/ic-5/.

Nutrient Digestion—the Absorb Max Difference

By the time most people are overweight, their digestive systems are no longer working properly for them. This poor digestion process can cause food intolerances as well as a lack of vital nutrient absorption. This stalls your ability to burn fat significantly as well... even if you are eating healthy foods.

Just how important is this? Well, according to a study conducted at Baylor Medical College, 98% of participants displayed significantly improved body composition and/or scale weight by adhering to one single dietary practice: removing foods from their diet for which they tested positive for intolerances. At the same time, a matched control group who followed a calorie-restricted diet alone actually GAINED weight. In other words, you must make sure that your digestive system is working optimally for you, in order to benefit from the vital nutrients you will be receiving from our *Taste of Life; An Intellectual Eating Plan*™, and the valuable supplements you take. The easiest and fastest way to do this is to take Absorbmax: waketheforkup.com/shop/biotrust-products/absorbmax/.

Promote Bowel Regularity, Reduce GI Inflammation, and Support Intestinal Health—Pro-X10™

Perhaps you yourself are already experiencing some of the more advanced **signs that your intestinal bacterial balance is beginning to spin out of control**, such as:

- Gas and bloating
- Constipation and/or diarrhea
- Fatigue
- Headaches
- Sugar cravings, especially for heavily refined carbs

In fact, there are more than 200 studies linking inadequate probiotic levels to more than 170 different health issues, including obesity and weight gain. Perhaps it is time for you to learn more about this unique supplement. Take it for a test drive here: waketheforkup.com/shop/biotrust-products/prox-10/.

In a nutshell, these are the best supplements YOU can take today to help spark the flame to your fat-burning furnace process. However, remember, supplements are exactly that; a supplemental approach to an existing sound Total Body Transformation System. Once you have this formula down, you should be well on your way to your best body ever. Please be sure to share your success story with us by sending your info to <u>waketheforkup@gmail.com</u>. Remember a picture is worth a thousand words... so please take before and after pictures. Who knows, maybe I will fly out to your location to interview YOU!

Note: Supplement Information and Research can all be found at <u>waketheforkup.biotrust.com/shop.asp</u>

IN CLOSING

"Your body is a finely tuned vehicle; give it good fuel, great movement and a clear precise direction, and it will take you places you only dreamed of."

—Gary Watson

In closing, I would like to remind YOU that you have all you need within you now to get the body, mind, and soul you have always dreamed of. Taking the right turn in the fork in the road is much easier than you think. In fact, when you follow my patented **Primary M.E. and the Power of Three**™ system, you will not fail. Remember, you must have a Map of this incredible journey that allows you to understand every turn in the road. **Your Mental Edge**™ is exactly this MAP.

You must have an exercise formula that is specifically designed to rev up your Seven Super Fat-Burning Hormones like a super sports car. Only **Dynamic Integrated Results-Based Training**™ can do this with ease in record time. You must learn to eat uniquely and specifically for YOUR Nutritional Metabolic Type. You must learn to eat within YOUR specific Intellectual Eating Window. It is the only way you will kill the cravings quickly and allow your body to instantly start burning fat as fuel. Of course, your **Taste of Life; An Intellectual Eating Plan**™ is exactly what you need. The system is truly groundbreaking and unlike anything you will hear about on the television, radio, or internet. This Total Body Transformation System is simple, yet specific. It is truly as easy as one, two, three, especially when I have laid out all the maps and directions in simple to follow instructions. I guarantee, no matter how many other programs you have tried in the past and have failed, your journey will be different this time. This time, you will become that lean fat-burning machine all of your friends will envy. Your vision, purpose, passion, and energy will be that of a superhuman. Take action today, and be sure to let me know how you are doing. I am eager to share your success story with the world. You can do it! Wouldn't NOW be a great time to start? waketheforkup.com/programs/

SELECTED BIBLIOGRAPHY

Adibi SA, (1976). Intestinal Phase of Protein Assimilation in Man. *Am. J. Clin. Nutr,* 29:205.

Ahima RS, et al. (2000). Leptin regulation of neuroendocrine systems. *Front Neuroendocrinolgy,* 21(3):263-307.

Ahima RS, Flier JS, (2000). Leptin. *Annu Rev Physiol,* 62:413-37. Review.

Ahmad F, Khan MM, Rastogi AK, Chaubey M, Kidwai JR. (1991). Effect of epicatechin on cAMP content, insulin release and conversion of proinsulin to insulin in immature and mature rat islets in vitro. *Indian J Exp Biol,* 29(6):516-20.

Akmal M, et al. (2009). The Effect of The ALCAT Test Diet Therapy for Food Sensitivity in Patient's With Obesity. *Middle East Journal of Family Medicine,* 7(3).

Aksungar, FB et al. (2007). Interleukin-6, C-reactive protein and biochemical parameters during prolonged intermittent fasting. *Ann Nutr Metab,* 51(1): 88-95.

Allison KC, et al. (2005). Neuroendocrine profiles associated with energy intake, sleep, and stress in the night eating syndrome. *Journal of Clinical Endocrinology and Metabolism,* 9, 6214-6217.

Anderson RA, et al. (2004). Isolation and characterization of polyphenol type-A polymers from cinnamon with insulin-like biological activity. *J Agric Food Chem,* 52(1):65-70.

Anson RM, et al. (2003). Intermittent fasting dissociates beneficial effects of dietary restriction on glucose metabolism and neuronal resistance to injury from calorie intake. *Proc Natl Acad Sci,* 100: 6216-20.

Aranceta J, Pérez-Rodrigo C, (2012). Recommended dietary reference intakes, nutritional goals and dietary guidelines for fat and fatty acids: a systematic review. *Br J Nutr,* 107 Suppl 2:S8-22.

Badmaev V, et al. (1999). Piperine, an Alkaloid Derived from Black Pepper, Increases Serum Response of Beta-Carotene During 14-days of Oral Beta-Carotene Supplementation. *Nutrition Research,* 19(3): 381-388

Belkacemi L, et al. (2012). Intermittent Fasting Modulation of the Diabetic Syndrome in Streptozotocin-Injected Rates. *Internal Journal of Endocrinology.*

Bellisle F, et al. (1997). Meal frequency and energy balance. *Br J Nutr,* 77 Suppl 1:S57-70.

Bellisle F, et al. (2004). Impact of the daily meal pattern on energy balance. *Scandinavian Journal of Nutrition,* 48(3): 114-118.

Bentley P, (2011). Not tonight, dear, I'm an insomniac: Lack of sleep kills men's sex drive, study finds. *The Daily Mail.* http://www.dailymail.co.uk/news/article-

Gary Watson

1393930/Lack-sleep-kills-mens-sex-drive-University-Chicago-study-finds.html

Beyondhealth.com. (2012). Free Report: The Roadmap to Supplements.

Bhasin S, Stoer TW, Berman N, Callegari C, Clevenger B, et al. (1996). The effects of supra- physiologic doses of testosterone on muscle size and strength in normal men. *N Engl J Med*, 335:1-7.

Blankson H, Stakkestad JA, Fagertun H, Thom E, Wadstein J, and Gudmundsen O, (2000). Conjugated linoleic acid reduces body fat mass in overweight and obese humans. *J Nutr*, 130: 2943-2948.

Boden G, et al. (1996). Effect of fasting on serum leptin in normal human subjects. *J Clin Endocrinol Metab*, 81(9):3419-23.

Bompa T, (1994). *Periodization of Strength: The New Wave in Strength Training*. Veritas Publications.

Borkman M, Campbell LV, Chisholm DJ, Storlien LH, (1991). Comparison of the Effects on Insulin Sensitivity of High Carbohydrate and High Fat Diets in Normal Subjects. *The Journal of Clinical Endocrinology & Metabolism*, 72(2), 432-437.

Bosello O, Zamboni M, (2000). Visceral obesity and metabolic syndrome. *Obesity reviews*, 1(1), 47-56

Boström P, et al. (2012). *A PGC1-α-dependent myokine that drives brown-fat-like development of white fat and*

thermogenesis. *Nature* 481: 463–468.
doi:10.1038/nature10777

Bosy-Westphal A, Kossel E, Goele K, et al. (2009). Contribution of individual organ mass loss to weight-loss associated decline in resting energy expenditure. *Am J
Clin Nutr*, 90:993–1001.

Boue, SM, et al. (2009). Identification of the potent phytoestrogen glycinol in elicited soybean (Glycine max). *Endocrinology, 150:2446-2453.*

Bowe WP, Logan AC, (2011). Acne vulgaris, probiotics and
the gut-brain-skin axis - back to the future? *Gut
Pathogens*, 3:1.

Bowles L, Kopelman P, (2001). Leptin: of mice and men? *J
Clin Pathol*, 54(1):1-3.

Buckley R, et al. (2004). Circulating triacylglycerol and apoE
levels in response to EPA and docosahexaenoic acid
supplementation in adult human subjects. *Br J Nutr*,
92(3):477-83.

Calder PC, Yaqoob P, (2009). Omega-3 polyunsaturated fatty
acids and human health outcomes. *Biofactors,*
35(3):266-72.

Camandola S, et al. (2003). Intermittent food deprivation
improves cardiovascular and neuroendocrine responses to stress in rats. *J Nutr*, 133(6): 1921-9.

Cameron JD, et al. (2009). Increased meal frequency does
not promote greater weight loss in subjects who were

prescribed an 8-week equi-energetic energy-restricted diet. *Br J Nutr*, 30:1-4.

Cani PD, Delzenne NM, (2010). Involvement of the gut microbiota in the development of low grade inflammation associated with obesity: focus on this neglected partner. *Acta Gastroenterol Belg*, 73(2):267-9.

Carey DG, Jenkins AB, Campbell LV, Freund J, Chisholm DJ, (1996). Abdominal fat and insulin resistance in normal and overweight women: direct measurements reveal a strong relationship in subjects at both low and high risk of NIDDM. *Diabetes*, 45(5), 633-638.

Carlson O, et al. (2007). Impact of Reduced Meal Frequency Without Caloric Restriction on Glucose Regulation in Healthy, Normal Weight Middle-Aged Men and Women. *Metabolism*, 56(12): 1729–1734.

Castro-Obregon S, (2010). The Discovery of Lysosomes and Autophagy. *Nature Education*, 3(9):49.

CDC. (2013). Insufficient Sleep Is a Public Health Epidemic. CDC.gov.

Chakravarthy M, Booth F, (2004). Eating, exercise, and "thrifty" genotypes: connecting the dots toward an evolutionary understanding of modern chronic diseases. *J Appl Physiol*, 96: 3-10.

Clark CD, Bassett B, Burge MR, (2003). Effects of kelp supplementation on thyroid function in euthyroid subjects. *Endocr Pract*, 9(5): 363-9.

Common GI Problems: Volume 1. (n.d.). *The American College of Gastroenterology*, Web.

ConsumerLab Independent Testing Group. Contamination and Other Problems Found in Fish Oil Supplements. August 22, 2012. *http://www.consumerlab.com/news/Review%20of %20Fish%20Oil%20and%20Omega-3%20Supplments%20by%20ConsumerLab.com/8_2 2_2012/*

Coral Calcium: Fact and Conjecture, (2006). *Natural Clinician*, 2006.

Davis, WJ, Wood, DT, Andrews, RG, Elkind, LM, and Davis, WB, (2008). Concurrent training enhances athletes' strength, muscle endurance, and other measures. *J Strength Cond Res,* 22(5): 1487-1502.

Deaton J, Dawson H, Davidson J, (2012). Prohydrolase with milk protein whey in a sports protein drink – a controlled study to evaluate efficacy. (unpublished research).

Del Piano M, et al. (2006). Probiotics: from research to consumer. *Dig Liver Dis*, 38 Suppl 2:S248-55.

Despres JP, (1992). Abdominal obesity as important component of insulin-resistance syndrome. *Nutrition,* 9(5): 452-459.

Deters AM, Schröder KR, Hensel A, (2005). Kiwi fruit (Actinidia chinensis L.) polysaccharides exert stimulating effects on cell proliferation via enhanced growth factor receptors, energy production, and collagen synthesis of human keratinocytes, fibroblasts, and skin equivalents. *J Cell Physiol,* 202(3):717-22.

Dharmadhikari SD, Patki VP, Dashputra PO, (1984). Study of mechanism of hypoglycaemia due to Pterocarpus marsupium. *Indian J Pharmacol,* 16, 61.

DiBaise JK, Zhang H, Crowell MD, Krajmalnik-Brown R, Decker GA, Rittmann BE, (2008). Gut microbiota and its possible relationship with obesity. *Mayo Clin Proc,* 83(4): 460-9.

Divi RL, et al. (1997). Anti-thyroid isoflavones from soybean: isolation, characterization, and mechanisms of action. *Biochem Pharmacol,* 54(10): 1087-96.

Doerge DR, et al. (2002). Inactivation of thyroid peroxidase by soy isoflavones, in vitro and in vivo. *J Chromatogr B Analyt Technol Biomed Life Sci,* 777(1-2): 269-79.

Doucet E, et al. (2000). Changes in energy expenditure and substrate oxidation resulting from weight loss in obese men and women: is there an important contribution of leptin? *J Clin Endocrinol Metab,* 85(4):1550-6.

Dubuc GR, Havel PJ, et al. (1998). Changes of serum leptin and endocrine and metabolic parameters after 7 days of energy rcotriction in men and women. *Metabolism,* 47(4):429-34.

Ehren J. et al. (2009). A Food-Grade Enzyme Preparation with Modest Gluten Detoxification Properties. *PLoS One,* 4(7): e6313.

Endocrine Society. (2011, June 7). Older age does not cause testosterone levels to decline in healthy men. *Science-Daily*. Retrieved December 2, 2014 from www.sciencedaily.com/releases/2011/06/110607121129.htm

Endocrine Society. (2012, June 23). Declining testosterone levels in men not part of normal aging. *ScienceDaily*. Retrieved December 2, 2014 from www.sciencedaily.com/releases/2012/06/120623144944.htm

Epel ES, et al. (2000). Stress and body shape: stress-induced cortisol secretion is consistently greater among women with central fat. *Psychosomatic Medicine*, 62(5), 623-632.

Farshchi HR, et al. (2005). Beneficial metabolic effects of regular meal frequency on dietary thermogenesis, insulin sensitivity, and fasting lipid profiles in healthy obese women. *Am J Clin Nutr*, (81):16 –24.

Fernie CE, et al. (2004). Relative absorption of conjugated linoleic acid as triacylglycerol, free fatty acid and ethyl ester in a functional food matrix. *European journal of lipid science and technology*, 106(6), 347-354.

Ferruccio S, et al. (2010). Acute exogenous TSH administration stimulates leptin secretion in vivo. *Eur J Endocrinol*, 163: 63-67.

Flachs P, et al. (2005). Polyunsaturated fatty acids of marine origin upregulate mitochondrial biogenesis and induce beta-oxidation in white fat. *Diabetologia*, 48(11): 2365-75.

Flachs P, et al. (2006). Polyunsaturated fatty acids of marine origin induce adiponectin in mice fed a high-fat diet. Diabetologia, 49(2): 394-7.

Gardner-Thorpe D, et al. (2003). Dietary supplements of soya flour lower serum testosterone concentrations and improve markers of oxidative stress in men. *Eur J Clin Nutr*, 57(1):100-6.

Garg A, Grundy SM, Unger RH, (1992). Comparison of effects of high and low carbohydrate diets on plasma lipoproteins and insulin sensitivity in patients with mild NIDDM. *Diabetes*, 41(10), 1278-1285.

Gaullier JM, et al. (2004). Conjugated linoleic acid supplementation for 1 yr reduces body fat mass in healthy overweight humans. *Am J Clin Nutr*, 79(6):1118-25.

Gladwell M, (2008). *Outliers: The Story of Success*. Little, Brown and Company.

Goodin S, et al. (2007). Clinical and biological activity of soy protein powder supplementation in healthy male volunteers. *Cancer Epidemiol Biomarkers Prev*, 16(4):829-33.

Goodman H, (2012). Natural "exercise" hormone transforms fat cells. Harvard Health Blog. http://www.health.harvard.edu/blog/natural-exercise-hormone-transforms-fat-cells-201206054851

Gratz SW, Mykkanen H, El-Nezami, HS, (2010). Probiotics and gut health: A special focus on liver diseases. *World J Gastroenterol*, 16(4): 403–410.

Greenway FL, Bray GA, Heber D, (1995). Topical fat reduction. *Obes Res*, 3 Suppl 4:561S-568S.

Grøntved A, et al. (2012). A Prospective Study of Weight Training and Risk of Type 2 Diabetes Mellitus in Men. *Archives of Internal Medicine.*

Guerra B, et al. (2011). Is sprint exercise a leptin signalling mimetic in human skeletal muscle? *J Appl Physiol*, 111(3): 715-25.

Halagappa VK, et al. (2007). Intermittent fasting and caloric restriction ameliorate age-related behavioral deficits in the triple-transgenic mouse model of Alzheimer's disease. *Neurobiol Dis*, 26(1): 212-20.

Hamosh M, et al. (1975). Pharyngeal lipase and digestion of dietary triglyceride in man. *J Clin Invest*, 55(5): 908–913.

Hannan JM, Ali L, Rokeya B, Khaleque J, Akhter M, Flatt PR, Abdel-Wahab YH, (2007). Soluble dietary fibre fraction of Trigonella foenum-graecum (fenugreek) seed improves glucose homeostasis in animal models of type 1 and type 2 diabetes by delaying carbohydrate digestion and absorption, and enhancing insulin action. *Br J Nutr*, 97(3): 514-21.

Harbige LS, (2003). Fatty acids, the immune response, and autoimmunity: a question of n-6 essentiality and the balance between n-6 and n-3. *Lipids*, 38(4): 323-41.

Harvie MN, Pegington M, Mattson MP, et al. (2005). The effects of intermittent or continuous energy restriction on weight loss and metabolic disease risk markers: a randomised trial in young overweight women. *International journal of obesity,* 35(5): 714-727.

He K, Liu K, Daviglus ML, et al. (2009). Associations of dietary long-chain n-3 polyunsaturated fatty acids and fish with biomarkers of inflammation and endothelial activation (from the Multi-Ethnic Study of Atherosclerosis [MESA]). *Am J Cardiol,* 103(9): 1238–1243.

Hermann R, Niebch G, Borbe HO, et al. (1996). Enantioselective pharmacokinetics and bioavailability of different racemic alpha-lipoic acid formulations in healthy volunteers. *Eur J Pharm Sci,* 4: 167-174.

Hlebowicz J, Darwiche G, Bjorgell O and Almer LO, (2007). Effect of cinnamon on postprandial blood glucose, gastric emptying, and satiety in healthy subjects. *Am J Clin Nutr,* 85: 1552-1556.

Hoffman JR, Ratamess NA, Kang J, Falvo MJ, Faigenbaum AD, (2006). Effect of protein intake on strength, body composition and endocrine changes in strength/power athletes. *Journal of the International society of Sports Nutrition,* 3(2): 12-18.

Högström M, et al. (2007). n-3 Fatty acids are positively associated with peak bone mineral density and bone accrual in healthy men: the NO2 Study. *Am J Clin Nutr,* 85(3): 803-7.

Hontecillas R, et al. (2009). Activation of PPAR γ and α by Punicic Acid Ameliorates Glucose Tolerance and Suppresses Obesity-Related Inflammation. *Journal of the American College of Nutrition,* 28(2): 184-195.

Hugot, JP, (2004). Inflammatory bowel disease: a complex group of genetic disorders. *Best Practice & Research Clinical Gastroenterology*, 18(3): 451-462.

Hussein GM, et al. (2011). Mate tea (Ilex paraguariensis) promotes satiety and body weight lowering in mice: involvement of glucagon-like peptide-1. *Biol Pharm Bull*, 34(12): 1849-55.

Indian Council of Medical Research (ICMR), (1998). Flexible dose open trial of Vijayasar (Pterocarpus marsupium) in cases of newly-diagnosed non-insulin-dependent diabetes mellitus. *Indian J Med Res*, 108: 253

Intermountain Medical Center. (2011). Study finds routine periodic fasting is good for health, and your heart. *ScienceDaily*.

Ishitani K, (1999). Calcium Absorption from the Ingestion of Coral-Derived Calcium by Humans. *J Nutr Sci Vitaminology*, 45(5), 509-517.

Islam, MA, Cheol-Heui Y, Yun-Jaie C, Chong-Su C, (2010). Microencapsulation of Live Probiotic Bacteria. *J. Microbiol. Biotechnol*, 20(10): 1367–1377.

Iwamoto T, Suzuki N, Tanabe K, Takeshita T, Hirofuji T, (2010). Effects of probiotic Lactobacillus salivarius WB21 on halitosis and oral health: an open-label pilot trial. *Oral Surg Oral Med Oral Pathol Oral Radiol Endod*, 110(2): 201-8.

Jacob S, Rett K, Henriksen EJ, Haring HU. (1999). Thioctic acid--effects on insulin sensitivity and glucose-metabolism. *Biofactors*, 10(2-3): 169-174.

James A, (2015). *The Wild Diet.* Penguin Group.

Jarvill-Taylor KJ, Anderson RA, Graves DJ, (2001). A hydroxychalcone derived from cinnamon functions as a mimetic for insulin in 3T3-L1 adipocytes. *J Am Coll Nutr,* 20(4):327-36.

Javed F, et al. (2010). Brain and high metabolic rate organ mass: contributions to resting energy expenditure beyond fat-free mass. *The American Journal of Clinical Nutrition, 91*(4), 907–912.

Jequier E, (2002). Leptin signaling, adiposity, and energy balance. *Ann NY Acad Sci,* 967: 379-88. Review.

Jevning R, Wilson AF, Davidson JM, (1978). Adrenocortical activity during meditation. *Hormones and Behavior,* 10(1): 54-60.

Johnson JB, et al. (2006). The effect on health of alternate day calorie restriction: eating less and more than needed on alternate days prolongs life. *Med Hypotheses,* 67(2): 209-11.

Johnson JB, et al. (2007). Alternate day calorie restriction improves clinical findings and reduces markers of oxidative stress and inflammation in overweight adults with moderate asthma. *Free Radic Biol Med,* 42(5): 665-74.

Jonas AJ, Butler IJ, (1989). Circumvention of defective neutral amino acid transport in Hartnup disease using tryptophan ethyl ester. *J Clin Invest,* 84(1): 200-4.

Jones PJ, et al. (1995). Meal frequency influences circulating hormone levels but not lipogenesis rates in humans. *Metabolism*, 44(2): 218-23.

Kaats GR, et al. (1996). The Short Term Efficacy of the AL-CAT Test of Food Sensitivities to Facilitate Changes in Body Composition and Self-Reported Disease Symptoms: A Randomized Controlled Study. *American Journal of Bariatric Medicine*.

Kadooka Y, et al. (2010). Regulation of abdominal adiposity by probiotics (Lactobacillus gasseri SBT2055) in adults with obese tendencies in a randomized controlled trial. *Eur J Clin Nutr*, 64(6): 636-43.

Katare RG, et al. (2009). Chronic intermittent fasting improves the survival following large myocardial ischemia by activation of BDNF/VEGF/PI3K signaling pathway. *J Mol Cell Cardiol*, 46(3): 405-1

Kennedy A, et al. (1997). The metabolic significance of leptin in humans: gender-based differences in relationship to adiposity, insulin sensitivity, and energy expenditure. *J Clin Endocrinol Metab*, 82(4): 1293-300.

Kessler DA, (2009). *The End of Overeating: Taking Control of the Insatiable American Appetite*. Rodale Inc.

Kirchgessner W, et al. (1987). Thermogenesis in humans after varying meal time frequency. *Ann Nutr Metab*, 31(2): 88-97.

Klein S, et al. (1990). Importance of blood glucose concentration in regulating lipolysis during fasting in humans. *Am J Physiol Endocrinol Metab*, 258: E32-E39.

Konarzewski M, Ksiazek A, (2013). Determinants of intra-specific variation in basal metabolic rate. *Journal of Comparative Physiology*, 183(1): 27-41.

Kong WJ, et al. (2009). Berberine reduces insulin resistance through protein kinase C-dependent up-regulation of insulin receptor expression. *Metabolism*, 58(1):109-19.

Kozubík A, Pospísil M, (1982). Protective effect of intermittent fasting on the mortality of gamma-irradiated mice. *Strahlentherapie*, 158(12): 734-8.

Kumari M, et al. (2009). Self-reported sleep duration and sleep disturbance are independently associated with cortisol secretion in the Whitehall II study. *The Journal of Clinical Endocrinology & Metabolism*, 94(12), 4801-4809.

Lawson LD, Hughes BG, (1988). Human absorption of fish oil fatty acids as triacylglycerols, free acids, or ethyl esters. *Biochem Biophys Res Commun*, 152(1): 328-35.

Levine AS, Billington CK, (1998). Do circulating leptin concentrations reflect body adiposity or energy flux? *Am J Clin Nutr*, 68: 761-762.

Leyer GJ, et al. (2009). Probiotic Effects on Cold and Influenza-LIke Symptom Incidence and Duration in Children. *Pediatrics*, 124: e172.

Lopez-Garcia E, Schulze MB, Manson JE, et al. (2004). Consumption of (n-3) fatty acids is related to plasma biomarkers of inflammation and endothelial activation in women. *J Nutr*, 134(7): 1806–1811.

Lye HS, et al. (2009). The Improvement of Hypertension by Probiotics: Effects on Cholesterol, Diabetes, Renin, and Phytoestrogens. *Int. J. Mol. Sci,* 10: 3755-3775.

Majamaa H, Isolauri E, (1997). Probiotics: a novel approach in the management of food allergy. *J Allergy Clin Immunol,* 99(2): 179-85.

Mandel AL, Breslin PAS, (2012). High endogenous salivary amylase activity is associated with improved glycemic homeostasis following starch ingestion in adults. *J Nutr,* 142(5): 853-8.

Mårin P, et al. (1992). Cortisol secretion in relation to body fat distribution in obese premenopausal women. *Metabolism*, 41(8): 882-886.

Mars M, et al. (2006). Fasting leptin and appetite responses induced by a 4-day 65%-energy-restricted diet. *Int J Obes*, 30(1): 122-8.

Martin B, Mattson MP, Maudsley S, (2006). Caloric restriction and intermittent fasting: two potential diets for successful brain aging. *Ageing Res Rev,* 5(3): 332-53.

Mattson M, (2008). Dietary factors, hormesis and health. *Ageing Res Rev*, 7(1): 43-8.

Mattson MP, Wan R, (2005). Beneficial effects of intermittent fasting and caloric restriction on the cardiovascular and cerebrovascular systems. *J Nutr Biochem,* 16(3): 129-37.

Mayanagi G, et al. (2009). Probiotic effects of orally administered Lactobacillus salivarius WB21-containing tablets on periodontopathic bacteria: a double-blinded, placebo-controlled, randomized clinical trial. *J Clin Periodontol,* 36(6): 506-13.

McAuley KA, et al. (2005). Comparison of high-fat and high-protein diets with a high-carbohydrate diet in insulin-resistant obese women. *Diabetologia,* 48(1): 8-16.

McFarland L, Bernasconi P, (1993). Saccharomyces boulardii: a review of an innovative biotherapeutic agent. *Microbial Ecology in Health and Disease,* 6: 157–71.

Mensink R, Katan, M, (1987). Effect of monounsaturated fatty acids versus complex carbohydrates on high-density lipoproteins in healthy men and women. *The Lancet, 329*(8525): 122-125.

Merat S, Casanada F, Sutphin M, Palinski W, Reaven PD, (1999). Western-type diets induce insulin resistance and hyperinsulinemia in LDL receptor-deficient mice but do not increase aortic atherosclerosis compared with normoinsulinemic mice in which similar plasma cholesterol levels are achieved by a fructose-rich diet. *Arteriosclerosis, thrombosis, and vascular biology,* 19(5), 1223-1230.

Mercola JM, (2012). Activating Your Brown Fat May Force Your Body to Burn 400-500 Extra Calories/Day. *Mercola.com.*

Mittendorfer B, et al. (2005). Protein Synthesis rates in human muscles: neither anatomical location nor fiber-type composition are major determinants. *J Physiol,* 563(1): 203-211

Miyawaki T, et al. (2002). Clinical implications of leptin and its potential humoral regulators in long-term low-calorie diet therapy for obese humans. *Eur J Clin Nutr,* 56(7):593-600.

Moosavi SA, et al. (2007). Evaluation of the effect of Islamic fasting on lung volumes and capacities in the healthy persons. *Saudi Med J,* 28(11): 1666-70.

Muller MJ, et al. (2011). Effect of Constitution on Mass of Individual Organs and Their Association with Metabolic Rate in Humans—A Detailed View on Allometric Scaling. *PLoS One,* 6(7): e22732.

Nedvidkova J, (1997). Leptin. *Cesk Fysiol,* 46(4): 182-8. Review.

Ngondi JL, Etoundi BC, Nyangono CB, Mbofung CM, Oben JE, (2009). IGOB131, a novel seed extract of the West African plant Irvingia gabonensis, significantly reduces body weight and improves metabolic parameters in overweight humans in a randomized double-blind placebo controlled investigation. *Lipids Health Dis,* 8:7

Nuria L, et al. (2007). Effects of milk supplementation with conjugated linoleic acid (isomers cis-9, trans-11 and trans-10, cis-12) on body composition and metabolic syndrome components. *Br J Nutr*, 98(4): 860-7.

Occhipinti MJ, et at. Weight Management, An Important Component of Health and Fitness. A Position Paper of the American Fitness Professionals and Associates (AFPA).

O'Connor A, (2013). How sleep loss adds to weight gain. *Nytimes.com*. http://well.blogs.ny-times.com/2013/08/06/how-sleep-loss-adds-to-weight-gain/?_r=1

O'Mara K, (2012). How Much Running Is Bad For Your Heart? *Competitor.com*.

Opperman M, et al. (2011). Analysis of omega-3 fatty acid content of South African fish oil supplements. *Cardiovasc J Afr*, 22(6): 324-9.

Parker DC, Rossman LG, VanderLaan EF, (1972). Persistence of Rhythmic Human Growth Hormone Release during Sleep in Fasted and Nonisocalorically Fed Normal Subjects. *Metabolism*, 21: 241

Pasiakos SM, McClung HL, McClung JP, Margolis LM, Andersen NE, Cloutier GJ, Pikosky MA, Rood JC, Fielding KA, Young AJ, (2011). Leucine-enriched essential amino acid supplementation during moderate steady state exercise enhances post exercise muscle protein synthesis. *Am J Clin Nutr*, 94(3): 809-18.

Penev PD, (2007). Association between sleep and morning testosterone levels in older men. *Sleep*, 30(4): 427-32.

Raff M, et al. (2009). Conjugated linoleic acids reduce body fat in healthy postmenopausal women. *J Nutr*, 139(7): 1347-52.

Rafferty, EP, et al. (2011). In Vitro and In Vivo Effects of Natural Putative Secretagogues of Glucagon-Like Peptide-1 (GLP-1). *Sci Pharm*, 79: 615–621.

Rayasam GV, et al. (2010). Identification of berberine as a novel agonist of fatty acid receptor GPR40. *Phytother Res*, 24(8): 1260-3.

Reinberg S, (2009). Millions of Americans don't get enough sleep. *US News and World Report*. http://health.us-news.com/health-news/family-health/sleep/articles/2009/10/29/millions-of-americans-dont-get-enough-sleep

Riserus U, et al. (2001). Conjugated linoleic acid (CLA) reduced abdominal adipose tissue in obese middle-aged men with signs of the metabolic syndrome: a randomised controlled trial. *International Journal of Obesity*, 25: 1129-1135

Riserus U, et al. (2002). Supplementation with conjugated linoleic acid causes isomer-dependent oxidative stress and elevated C-reactive protein: a potential link to fatty acid-induced insulin resistance. *Circulation*, 106: 1925–9.

Roth SM, (2006). Why does lactic acid build up in muscles? And why does it cause soreness? *Scientific American*.

Gary Watson

http://www.scientificamerican.com/article/why-does-lactic-acid-buil/

Rubio-Rodríguez N, et al. (2012). Supercritical fluid extraction of fish oil from fish by-products: A comparison with other extraction methods. *Journal of Food Engineering*, 109(2): 238-248.

Ruby BC, Gaskill SE, Slivka D, Harger SG, (2005). The addition of fenugreek extract (Trigonella foenum-graecum) to glucose feeding increases muscle glycogen resynthesis after exercise. *Amino Acids.* 28(1): 71-6.

Safdie FM, et al. (2009). Fasting and cancer treatment in humans: A case series report. *Aging*.

Sandberg AS, Andersson H, (1988). Effect of Dietary Phytase on the Digestion of Phytate in the Stomach and Small Intestine of Humans. *Jn Nutrition*, 118(4): 469-73.

Sathyapalan T, et al. (2011). The effect of soy phytoestrogen supplementation on thyroid status and cardiovascular risk markers in patients with subclinical hypothyroidism: a randomized, double-blind, crossover study. *J Clin Endocrinol Metab,* 96(5): 1442-9.

Sawhney PL, Seshadri TR, (1956). Special chemical components of commercial woods and related plant materials: Part IV - Phenolic components of some Pterocarpus species. *Journal of Science in India*, 15C: 154.

Schoenfeld B, (2010). The Mechanisms of Muscle Hypertrophy and Their Application to Resistance Training. *Journal of Strength and Conditioning Research*, 24(10): 2857-2872.

Schwellenbach LJ, et al. (2006). The triglyceride-lowering effects of a modest dose of docosahexaenoic acid alone versus in combination with low dose eicosapentaenoic acid in patients with coronary artery disease and elevated triglycerides. *J Am Coll Nutr*, 25(6): 480-5.

Selvam R, et al. (2009). Effect of Bacillus subtilis PB6, a natural probiotic on colon mucosal inflammation and plasma cytokines levels in inflammatory bowel disease. *Indian J Biochem Biophys*, 46(1): 79-85.

Serrano Rios M, et al. (1990). Nocturnal Growth Hormone Surges in Type 1 Diabetes Mellitus are Both Sleep and Glycemia Dependant: Assessment under Continuous Sleep Monitoring. *Diabetes Res Clin Pract*, 10: 1

Siegel I, et al. (1998). Effects of short-term dietary restriction on survival of mammary ascites tumor-bearing rats. *Cancer Invest.*

Siepmann T, et al. (2011). Hypogonadism and erectile dysfunction associated with soy product consumption. *Nutrition,* 27(7-8): 859-62.

Siff M, (2003). *Facts and Fallacies of Fitness.* M.C. Siff.

Sijben JW, Calder PC, (2007). Differential immunomodulation with long-chain n-3 PUFA in health and chronic disease. *Proc Nutr Soc*, 66(2): 237-59.

Silk DBA, Grimble GK, Rees RG, (1985). Protein digestion and amino acid and peptide absorption. *Proceedings of the Nutrition Society,* 44: 63-72.

Simopoulos AP, (2002). Omega-3 fatty acids in inflammation and autoimmune diseases. *J Am Coll Nutr*,
21(6):495-505.

Simopoulos AP, (2008). The importance of the omega-
6/omega-3 fatty acid ratio in cardiovascular disease
and other chronic diseases. *Exp Biol Med*, 233(6):
674-88.

Singh T, Newman AB, (2011). Inflammatory markers in population studies of aging. *Ageing Res Rev*, 10(3): 319–
329

Smedman A, Vessby B. (2001). Conjugated linoleic acid supplementation in humans--metabolic effects. *Lipids*,
36(8): 773-81.

Smeets AJ, et al. (2008). Acute effects on metabolism and
appetite profile of one meal difference in the lower
range of meal frequency. *British Journal of Nutrition*
(99): 1316–1321.
Snitker S, et al. (2009). Effects of novel capsinoid treatment
on fatness and energy metabolism in humans: possible pharmacogenetic implications. *Am J Clin Nutr*,
89(1): 45-50.

Snyder A, (2007). New Year, New Understanding of How
Fasting Affects the Brain. *Scientific American.*

SourceOne Global Partners. (2012). VESIsorb® Delivery
System. *Source-1-Global.com.*

Stanford University Medical Center. (2004, December 9).
Stanford Study Links Obesity To Hormonal Changes

From Lack Of Sleep. *ScienceDaily*. Retrieved December 2, 2014 from www.sciencedaily.com/releases/2004/12/041206194344.htm

Steinhoff U, (2005). Who controls the crowd? New findings and old questions about the intestinal microflora. *Immunol. Lett,* 99(1): 12–6.

Stonehouse W, et al. (2013). DHA supplementation improved both memory and reaction time in healthy young adults: a randomized controlled trial. *Am J Clin Nutr*, 97(5): 1134-43.

Stote KS, et al. (2007). A controlled trial of reduced meal frequency without caloric restriction in healthy, normal-weight, middle-aged adults. *American Journal of Clinical Nutrition*, 85(4): 981-988.

Sullivan A, Nord CE, Evengård B, (2009). Effect of supplement with lactic-acid producing bacteria on fatigue and physical activity in patients with chronic fatigue syndrome. *Nutrition Journal,* 8: 4.

Taheri S, Lin L, Austin D, Young T, Mignot E, (2004). Short Sleep Duration Is Associated with Reduced Leptin, Elevated Ghrelin, and Increased Body Mass Index. Froguel P, ed. *PLoS Medicine,* 1(3): e62.

Tam CS, et al. (2012). Brown Adipose Tissue. *Circulation*, 125: 2782-2791

Tanaka M, et al. (2009). Isoflavone supplements stimulated the production of serum equol and decreased the serum dihydrotestosterone levels in healthy male volunteers. *Prostate Cancer Prostatic Dis*, 12(3): 247-52.

Taussig SJ, Batkin S, (1988). Bromelain, the enzyme complex of pineapple (ananascomosus) and its clinical application. An update. *J Ethnopharmacol.* 22(2): 191-203.

Taylor MA, et al. (2001). Compared with nibbling, neither gorging nor a morning fast affect short-term energy balance in obese patients in a chamber calorimeter. *International Journal of Obesity,* 25: 519-528

The International Fish Oil Standards Program. (2012). Fact Sheet: Fish Oil Contaminants & Your Health.

The University of Chicago Medicine. (2011). Sleep loss lowers testosterone in healthy young men. *uchospitals.edu.* http://www.uchospitals.edu/news/2011/20110531-sleep.html

Thom E, et al. (2001). Conjugated Linoleic Acid Reduces Body Fat in Healthy Exercising Humans. *Journal of International Medical Research,* 29: 392

Turek VF, et al. (2010). Mechanisms of amylin/leptin synergy in rodent models. *Endocrinology,* 151(1): 143-52.

Van Dijk G, (2001). The role of leptin in regulation of energy balance and adiposity. *J Neuroendocrinol,* 13(10):913-21.

Varady K, Hellerstein MK, (2007). Alternate-day fasting and chronic disease prevention: a review of human and animal trials. *Am J Clin Nutr,* 86(1): 7-13.

Varady KA, et al. (2008). Modified alternate-day fasting regimens reduce cell proliferation rates to a similar extent as daily calorie restriction in mice. *FASEB J*, 22(6): 2090-6.

Venket Rao A, et al. (2009). A randomized, double-blind, placebo-controlled pilot study of a probiotic in emotional symptoms of chronic fatigue syndrome. *Gut Pathogens* 1:6

Verboeket-van de Venne WP, Westerterp KR, (1991). Influence of the feeding frequency on nutrient utilization in man: consequences for energy metabolism. *Eur J Clin Nutr*, 45(3): 161-9.

Vgontzas AN, et al. (2000). Chronic Systemic Inflammation in Overweight and Obese Adults. *AMA*, 283(17): 2235-2236.

Volek JS, et al. (2002). Body composition and hormonal responses to a carbohydrate-restricted diet. *Metabolism*, 51(7): 864-870.

Vroegrijk IO, et al. (2011). Pomegranate seed oil, a rich source of punicic acid, prevents diet-induced obesity and insulin resistance in mice. *Food and Chemical Toxicology*, 49(6): 1426-1430.

Wang Z, Ying Z, Bosy-Westphal A, et al. (2010). Specific metabolic rates of major organs and tissues across adulthood: evaluation by mechanistic model of resting energy expenditure. *Am J Clin Nutr*, 92: 1369–1377.

Wang Z, Ying Z, Bosy-Westphal A, et al. (2011). Evaluation of specific metabolic rates of major organs and tissues: comparison between men and women. *Am J Hum Biol*, 23: 333–338.

Warner K, et al. (2013). Oceana Study Reveals Seafood Fraud Nationwide. *Oceana Consumer Advocacy Group.* *http://oceana.org/sites/default/files/National_Seaf ood_Fraud_Testing_Results_FINAL.pdf*

Weigle DS, et al. (1997). Effect of fasting, refeeding, and dietary fat restriction on plasma leptin levels. *J Clin Endocrinol Metab*, 82(2): 561-5.

Weldon SM, et al. (2007). Docosahexaenoic acid induces an anti-inflammatory profile in lipopolysaccharide-stimulated human THP-1 macrophages more effectively than eicosapentaenoic acid. *J Nutr Biochem*, 18(4): 250-8.

Westerterp-Plantenga MS, (2010). Green tea catechins, caffeine and body-weight regulation. *Physiol Behav*, 100(1): 42-6.

Whiteman H, (2014). Shivering 'as good as exercise' for producing brown fat. *Medical News Today.* http://www.medicalnewstoday.com/articles/272258.php

Wikipedia. (2014). Night eating syndrome. Wikipedia.com. http://en.wikipedia.org/wiki/Night_eating_syndrome

Wisse BE, et al. (1999). Effect of prolonged moderate and severe energy restriction and refeeding on plasma leptin concentrations in obese women. *Am J Clin Nutr*, 70(3): 321-30.

Wolcott W, Fahey T, (2002). *The Metabolic Typing Diet.* Crown Publishing Group.

Yang CY, et al. (2010). Anti-diabetic effects of Panax noto-ginseng saponins and its major anti-hyperglycemic components. *J Ethnopharmacol,* 130(2): 231-6.

Yang S. (2005). Fasting every other day, while cutting few calories, may reduce cancer risk. Univ of California release, 2005-03-14.

Yin J, Xinga H, Ye J, (2008). Efficacy of Berberine in Patients with Type 2 Diabetes. *Metabolism,* 57(5): 712–717.

Zampelas A, et al. (2005). Fish consumption among healthy adults is associated with decreased levels of inflammatory markers related to cardiovascular disease: the ATTICA study. *J Am Coll Cardiol,* 46(1): 120–124.

Zargar A, Ito, MK, (2011). Long chain omega-3 dietary supplements: a review of the National Library of Medicine Herbal Supplement Database. *Metab Syndr Relat Disord,* 9(4): 255-71.

Zatsiorsky V, Kraemer WJ, (2006). *Science and Practice of Strength Training* (2nd ed). Human Kinetics.

Zhang H, et al. (2010). Berberine lowers blood glucose in type 2 diabetes mellitus patients through increasing insulin receptor expression. *Metabolism,* 59(2): 285-92.

Zimmet P, (1996). Serum leptin concentration, obesity, and insulin resistance in Western Samoans: cross sectional study. *BMJ,* 313(7063): 965-9.

Made in the USA
Middletown, DE
14 January 2019